Behind the Mask
of Moebius Syndrome

T0055257

Behind the Mask of Moebius Syndrome

A Memoir

CRISTINA FARAGLI

Foreword by RONALD M. ZUKER, M.D.

McFarland & Company, Inc., Publishers
Jefferson, North Carolina

LIBRARY OF CONGRESS CATALOGUING-IN-PUBLICATION DATA

Names: Faragli, Cristina, 1970– author.
Title: Behind the mask of moebius syndrome : a memoir / Cristina
     Faragli ; foreword by Ronald M. Zuker, M.D.
Description: Jefferson, N.C. : McFarland & Company, Inc., Publishers,
     2016. | Includes index.
Identifiers: LCCN 2016005935 | ISBN 9780786498383 (softcover :
     acid free paper) ∞
Subjects: LCSH: Faragli, Cristina, 1970– —Health. | Facial paralysis—
     Patients—Biography. | Facial nerve—Diseases.
Classification: LCC RC418 .F36 2016 | DDC 616.8/42092—dc23
LC record available at http://lccn.loc.gov/2016005935

BRITISH LIBRARY CATALOGUING DATA ARE AVAILABLE

ISBN (print) 978-0-7864-9838-3
ISBN (ebook) 978-1-4766-2295-8

© 2016 Cristina Faragli. All rights reserved

*No part of this book may be reproduced or transmitted in any form
or by any means, electronic or mechanical, including photocopying
or recording, or by any information storage and retrieval system,
without permission in writing from the publisher.*

Front cover image: Cristina Faragli, winter 1979 (author)

Printed in the United States of America

McFarland & Company, Inc., Publishers
  Box 611, Jefferson, North Carolina 28640
  www.mcfarlandpub.com

To Roberto, my one and only love, my better half. And for my parents. If they could read this book, they would realize that they had done a good job.

Table of Contents

Acknowledgments

Here I am, at the end of this incredible voyage—at least from my humble point of view.

When my husband suggested that I put my whole life on paper, a few months before I underwent smile surgery, at first I thought he was kidding. I continued to think so even after the third or fourth time he insisted. Then I started to suspect he was talking seriously, and most of all that he *was* deadly serious about it. I timidly objected that I hadn't taken a pen in hand since high school. About twenty years, more or less. Nonsense. What is more, this was not about putting together something for a class assignment. This was—a book about my life!? How could he think that I might be able to do it?

He insisted. When he wants, he can be stubborn. And petulant, too. But always immensely adorable. How could I say no? Okay, rhetorical question, let's try again. How could I ever deny him anything? Uhm, there is no way out, rhetoric haunts me. Anyway, after some quiet grumbling I gave up, and one spring day in 2013 I sat before a white computer screen.

The first sentences came out with difficulty, stumbling all the time. I wrote and rewrote, corrected and revised them. This, of course, gave me an excuse to get up from my chair, run to my husband and complain. The holy man patiently listened to that first outburst (kind of "I-can't-do-that-I-just-cannot" repeated over and over) and many more after that.

Then, day after day, my story took shape, and sentences were beginning to flow more naturally, so much so that I was literally glued to that chair—which I had initially hated so much—for whole nights. I wrote the final word, "*Petalùda*" (butterfly, in Greek), only a few days before leaving for Parma to face surgery.

I don't know if this book will speak to the heart of those people who, like me, have had to deal with any kind of *diversity*. I tried to speak to them because I wanted so much that the awareness and self-confidence which grew in me over the years could reach young souls, like Alice, who still have such a long road ahead. We are *normal* people, just like the others and sometimes even more so. It took me 30 years to figure that out, but I hope that this message will arrive in time for many of them. In time to save time. I don't know whether I will reach my goal, but one thing is for sure. This book has at least one merit: it definitely has had a cathartic function for me and prepared me properly for the biggest challenge that awaited me.

So, thank you Rob, you tireless, insistent, incredible love of my life. The first "thank you," and millions more with it, is for you. Without your constant support, this book would have never come to life.

The second "thank you," for obvious reasons, goes to Renzo De Grandi, president of A.I.S.Mo., and his wonderful family, without whom I would never have reached today's results. Thank you, Renzo, Caterina, Giulia, Aunt Pina, for your courage, determination, stubbornness and love. You made my life—and those of countless others—take a better direction, and there will never be appropriate words to show my gratitude towards you.

Thanks also to Dr. Ronald Zuker, who has dedicated his life to the study of the syndrome and who finally perfected "smile surgery," a technique that was unthinkable until the nineties. Ronald gave to so many people the smile they always wished for, and we will be all eternally grateful to him for that.

Thanks to Dr. Bernardo Bianchi and his team at the maxillofacial department at Parma Hospital, who have done a wonderful job on me and on many others, introducing Dr. Zuker's "smile surgery" into Italy.

An enormous thank you goes also to Daniela at A.I.S.Mo. Without that phone conversation we had, my dear, I would have not been able to decide whether to undergo surgery or not. You have been decisive in this. And Aunt Pina knows something about that too, so thank you from the bottom of my hear, sweet Pina.

Thanks also to Vicki McCarrel of the Moebius Syndrome Foundation in the United States, and to all the associations dedicated to the syndrome throughout the world. There are many! They are doing a great job! A special smile goes to you all.

Thanks very much to those who read the manuscript and helped me in many ways: Alberto Pezzotta, who read the very first Italian draft and kindly assisted me with feedback and suggestions; Mark Thompson Ashworth and Pete Tombs, who helped me with part of the translation, thoroughly revised the English version and corrected all my many errors, all with incredible patience and incomparable kindness; and Antonio Bosi, who fixed my old photographs. My love goes to you all!

And now a special acknowledgment to a person who, for better or for worse, has changed my life. I am talking about you, Jorgos. If I think about it, you saved my life not once but twice: the first time when we got together, the second when we broke up. Therefore, you mean twice as much to me, even if it is just because of that. I want to tell you in your language as well, since in Greek there is no difference between "I care about you" and "I love you." I am sure you will choose the right one. *S'a-gapò*.

Thanks to my dear, wonderful friends who read this work before it was published, even though they knew very well my adventures and misfortunes, because they were by my side too, almost always. A few people have a special part in my life: Antonella, Iko, Barbara, Lorenza, Rosanna, Eleonora, Elisa (Nicola, don't be jealous, this is time for girls), Ilaria, Simona (Tommy, I know you'll understand), and the most recent one, Alice.

And let's not forget the boys: Nicola, Tommaso, Alberto, Ferdinando, Lele, Stratos, Ferro, Max, Edu, Luca, Enrico, Andrea, Francesco—you were all wonderful, and I mean it!

And then, and then ... a very special acknowledgment goes to you, my dearest Ioanna and Vasilis, friends lost and found after 20 years. Time has not changed any of the feelings that bound us together. Indeed, it has multiplied the strength of our mutual affection. You were the first to read this story, and you were fantastic in commenting on every single paragraph. You have read, studied, dissected it like no other ever will, and all because you care about me so much, as I had always been a part of your life.

I adore you, don't ever forget it!

Last but not least, thanks to my family. A sweet thought goes to my mother and father, to whom also this book is dedicated. I love you so very much, and I hope that you will at least receive one billionth of that love where you are now. It would be sufficient. Thanks also to my wonderful, irreplaceable sisters. The Sisters. Always in the plural, two entities in one. I can never thank you enough for being there for me, ALWAYS. Thanks also to my incredible niece, Elena, and nephew, Samuele, and to my sweet in-laws, Roma and Giancarlo. All of you had a part in my current happiness.

Have I forgotten anyone? No doubt about that...

So, to make no mistake, I would like to thank everyone I have met even once in my life, from the child who first pointed his fat little finger at me to the one I met yesterday at the movies who turned to me and said, "You are the nice lady from the opticians'!" All, all, all of you, good and bad, pleasant and unpleasant, you have helped in building my actual self, the self I like so much.

One last thing. Thanks, Rob. Thank you for simply being in this world.

Foreword
by Ronald M. Zuker, M.D.

There are so many facets to Moebius syndrome. It is a complex condition with complex consequences.

I became involved many years ago through my work with facial paralysis, a common component of Moebius syndrome. There were only suboptimal treatments, poor surgical outcomes and shattered lives following surgical interventions. The early days of microsurgery (in the 1970s and 1980s) offered an opportunity for innovation and improvement in surgical outcomes. And so it was that I entered the field, trying to create new surgical procedures that would allow the Moebius syndrome patient to smile.

Smile surgery consists of relocating a muscle from the thigh to the face, carefully positioning it and, through the aid of the operating microscope, micro-instruments and microsutures, giving it a new blood supply and nerve connection.

The people I encountered on this surgical journey were remarkable. The patients showed amazing courage in dealing with the condition, getting on with their lives and becoming productive members of society. But also they exhibited an incredible sensitivity that parallels their courage in understanding behavior patterns and the feelings of others. The families were so close knit and supportive. To work with these families has been an honor. To see the patients grow up, marry, have children of their own, and work in the public arena has been most gratifying. They are a remarkable group of individuals, each with stories that need to be heard, need to be reflected upon and need to lead us to adjust our lives accordingly.

This is Cristina's story. Enjoy.

Ronald M. Zuker, M.D., FRCSC, is a pediatric reconstructive microsurgeon who has spent his career treating children at the Hospital for Sick Children in Toronto. His focus is on facial reanimation with innovative nerve and muscle transplants. He is also a professor of surgery at the University of Toronto.

1

Preface

Moebius syndrome is a rare congenital neurological disorder that strikes 2 to 20 newborn children for each million people: its main characteristic is permanent facial paralysis caused by the underdevelopment of several cranial nerves. In Italy, my country, there are about 300 known cases as of today.

People with Moebius syndrome cannot grimace, frown, wrinkle their noses, and often cannot even close or move their eyes from side to side. Above all, they cannot smile. All this turns their faces into expressionless masks. They are reduced to motionless surfaces, incapable of communicating feelings or sensations. This causes many limitations and problems, especially in everyday relationships.

Being affected by Moebius Syndrome means having to face curious and inquisitive looks, as well as the sometimes cruel reaction on the part of those who cannot accept other people's "diversity." It means having to deal with little obstacles and misunderstandings, which can often cause considerable psychological difficulties. It means having to get used to a different kind of life, in which even the most insignificant actions—like eating, or smiling—turn into a problem. All this can compromise a full integration into society.

I have been affected by Moebius Syndrome since birth, although at first I did not even know its name. My path towards finding a solution to this condition, which was almost totally unheard of in Italy at that time, was very complicated. It took a long, long time before I could finally give a name to the syndrome I was affected by—the first ten years of my life. However, knowing its name did not in itself bring any solution.

Moebius syndrome cannot be cured, but its effects can be partially limited, by way of surgery. Throughout the years, I have undergone a number of operations and medical treatments to at least partially ameliorate my situation. Finally, after several tentative, ill-fated efforts, in 2013 I underwent the so-called smile surgery. It was perfected by a Canadian plastic surgeon, Dr. Ronald Zuker, and it is aimed at allowing Moebius Syndrome patients to be finally able to smile.

I have told my whole life story in this book. All that I describe in these pages belongs to me, down to the slightest detail. I chose to bare myself completely, putting on paper all the feelings and emotions that accompanied me since birth. I tried to recall every single step in my own experience regarding Moebius Syndrome: the difficulties in everyday life, in my family and in my relationships with the opposite sex, as well as the medical treatments and the daily battles to convey my feelings when dealing with other people.

My story has a happy ending. In spite of everything I managed to reach a happy life, and I don't reject any of it, not even the most painful and frustrating moments. They were also part of making me who I am today. Still, I feel that my story can be helpful to those who are undergoing difficulties of any kind, either of a physical or a character nature, and somehow give them a little hope. Sometimes we all feel detached from the rest of the world, as if we were unable to relate to others, hopelessly trapped behind a mask.

Readers may get in touch with me at krysty1970@libero.it.

ONE

In the Cocoon

Awakening

"Cristina, open your eyes."

No, I don't want to. Leave me alone. I'm sleepy. It's nice here, peaceful and quiet, and I don't feel like listening to you.

"Cristina, do you hear me? Come on, open your eyes, it's all over, you must wake up now."

No, I'm tired. Leave me alone. I'm exhausted, worn out, spent. I don't even have the strength to speak. I don't think I'll answer. I think I'll ignore you. And who are you, by the way? Is that you, Mom? No, it can't be. My mom has been gone for many years now—too many. So who are you, then? How do you know my name? And why am I lying here in a strange bed, in a place I'm not familiar with?

There is so much light—I can even feel it through my closed eyelids—and pungent smells, and sounds that echo from near and far at the same time. It is all so strange, so unusual. And I'm thirsty; I'm so thirsty.

"Cristina, everything went just fine. We are taking you back to your room now. But you must wake up. Now."

Oh, yes, of course. Now I'm beginning to understand. My mind clears up moment by moment; the neurons do their duty and reconnect gradually with one another. Images take shape and find their place in a sequence that becomes clearer and clearer as it progresses. Then finally comes the memory, the awareness.

I'm in a hospital, and somebody I don't know—a female—is trying to get me out of the stupor of general anesthesia—a nurse, probably.

Oh well, give me just a little more time, my dear faceless companion, be patient. It feels so good here, halfway between sleep and waking. It is

5

all so quiet and safe; it's like a refuge. A womb—no, wait. A cocoon. Here's what it is like: a warm, cozy cocoon. And I have no desire to leave it.

Wait one more second, please. I need to rest a little more. I am so tired, you know, I fought for so long that I need a break, a moment of self-reflection. Indeed, I would really like to share some time with you, tell you who I am, and revisit the long journey that brought me here to this hospital bed. Don't rush me, please, so I can let the memories come flooding back.

I think I deserved this break, I really do. And, you know, if you have patience, I have the feeling you might like my story.

My name is Cristina, but I guess you already know that, since you have been calling my name for a while in an attempt to snap me out of this pleasant post-surgery drowsiness. By the way, what is your name? Oh, wait. Let me pick one, will you? I think I'll call you Nancy—Nancy like the girl sitting next to me during my first plane flight. I was alone, inexperienced, and very nervous, and she guessed it. She did not know me at all, and yet she sensed I was in trouble. So she started talking to me, suggesting I close my eyes and take a deep breath before takeoff. I clung to her words as if they were a life jacket, kept my eyes shut until she told me it was safe to open them again, and then I found her sweet smile waiting for me, a smile I would never forget.

Nancy is also the name of the French city where I underwent surgery, many years ago. Back then I was as sleepy as I am now, but no one bothered to gently shake me as you are doing. They simply waited until I opened my eyes on my own, whenever I felt like it. You know what was the first thing I saw when I finally woke up?

My mother. Of course. Who else could it be if not the person who loved me more than anyone else in the world? That's why earlier on I had thought—hoped—that you were her, but it was just a moment, that fraction of a second that always comes before you reconnect with reality.

Do not think my life was full of hospital visits and painful surgery, Nancy. It would be unfair to let you think that. This is only the third time I have put my life in the hands of a surgeon, and in forty years of existence that's not so many. I am well aware that there are people who have suffered much more than me in a much shorter period of time, but, you see, in my case one never knows what advantages or disadvantages will follow after all the hassle, the pain, the suffering.

To put your fate in the hands of a doctor, someone whom you have seen only a couple of times at most, always causes me a certain uneasiness. Nevertheless, now it was really necessary: the passage of time is unforgiving to everyone, and to me in particular. I had to make a final decision, a radical and brave one. I can only hope that this time, unlike in the past, it was worth it.

I am a living question mark, a puzzle that you cannot fully decipher.

I came into this world affected by a syndrome that was tentatively given a name only ten years after my birth. Before that, none of the doctors I met had ever come across a case like mine. I learned very early on to give the proper meaning to a word that I would hear repeated over and over again in the coming years: *rarity*.

Sure, it's true; each of us is unique and inimitable in our own way. I look at my hands, I think of my fingerprints, and the way each human being is different and recognizable in diversity.

But I am not just a particular human being. I am a *rarity*. I always associated this funny term with a sense of unease, discomfort, and loneliness. It is not pleasant being a rarity. It does not bring anything good.

Rarity frightens others.

Rarity attracts curious glances.

Rarity brings embarrassing questions.

Rarity arouses people's hostility and amplifies their dark side.

Rarity turns you into an island and abandons you in the midst of an ocean of ignorance, far away from everyone else.

I did not choose to be different, nor did I ask for any special regard. It just happened—to me, one case among millions of people—without any specific reason. Furthermore, the very fact of not knowing why all this started, and especially how it could be possible, always made my life quite frustrating: not being able to blame anyone or anything does not allow you to vent the anger you have inside, and you do have a lot of anger in you. If you are unable to channel it, it could even be dangerous. Over the years, fortunately, I have given up looking for a scapegoat. It wouldn't have changed my situation in any case, not in the least.

Ever since I was born, I wanted to make things clear.

There is no getting around it, Nancy, and it's best you know this right now: one of the things that has accompanied me for a lifetime is my trademark laziness.

If you asked me to walk even a couple of steps more than was strictly necessary, I'd stop in the middle of the road as if I were at a red traffic light. If I had to get up from a comfortable chair to hand you something, I'd most certainly tell you that I couldn't because, unfortunately, a cramp is stiffening my leg right now. If ... well, you get the picture.

I have felt like a sloth inside, ever since I was lying in the warmth of my mother's womb. I did not want to come into this world. And so, almost twenty days after my scheduled birth date, the doctors decided to force me out with a Caesarean section. Otherwise, there would have been big problems after birth. Meanwhile, inside that comfortable and quiet shelter, I had reached the considerable weight of eleven pounds and a bit. No one has ever been able to tell me how much that "bit" actually was. There are several stories about it, all of them underlined by the recollection that the birth was by no means easy, because of my size.

To get me out of my peaceful slumber, the doctors were forced to use a tool whose name I have always been scared of, and which still today sends a chill down my spine every time I utter it: forceps. This particular object, in my early years, became a focus of interest on the part of those who were searching for the origins of my problem and attempting to find a reason for my condition. Personally, I never believed that a mere mechanical instrument might have been able to cause so much damage. It always seemed to me a rather banal explanation for everything that came afterward. However, the doctors that examined me did not think the same way I did. It was as if they were trying to fix on some obscure circumstance, even the most fragile and unlikely, to be able to find an answer. Their bewilderment in facing a case like mine was utterly under-standable, anyway. I was a real *rarity*.

During the first few hours after birth, I began to create a number of difficulties, starting with problem number one: breast-feeding. The fact that I could not feed from my mother's breast might have seemed a rather common occurrence at first: so many newborn babies do without it. It was not a novelty. The real oddity was that I was not even interested in sucking milk from a normal bottle. And yes, that was bizarre. That was really weird. A *rarity*. The first in a long, long series of rarities.

Sometimes I think that nature endowed me with a few extra pounds at birth in order to overcome the bewilderment of those early days, when nobody could understand the reason why I did not want to feed. Day after day, I kept rejecting food, and the perplexities of those who took care of me were rising, in tandem with the descent of my own weight. The syn-drome was already at work, ready to challenge me and whoever was around me. It was the first of many battles. The syndrome, which would be devoid of a name for many years, was already putting a spoke in my wheels.

I really think it would have won had not my mother been such a stub-born woman and so full of initiative. She was a capable and determined person—a fighter. I always feel emotional when I think of all the tricks and stratagems that she adopted in order to feed me. I ponder on how hard it was to understand the reason for my lack of appetite, and how depressing to see so many attempts fail.

Actually, I was hungry—very hungry. And I cried out my impatience and indignation at the top of my voice, thus making it all the more frustrating, all the more unbearable for those around me. But how could they understand? How could they imagine that my problem was a congenital one? How could they help a newborn baby who could not use most of her facial muscles?

I came into this world with a severe form of facial paralysis. It involved the right side of my face and, in a subtler but still relevant form, the left one as well. This meant that I could not, and I still cannot, do all the things that a normal person does with such muscles—even the most common ones.

I cannot frown when I am puzzled. I cannot squeeze my eyes tightly closed when I am scared. I cannot snort if I am irritated. I cannot wrinkle my nose if I am upset.

And above all, I cannot smile when I am happy. This I always missed more than anything else. A smile can communicate happiness, harmony, and love. A smile can convey understanding, joy, and complicity.

I was robbed of the ability to get straight to other people's hearts. I was deprived of the ability to empathize with them, and communicate a sense of understanding. My feelings were captured and locked into a box—a body—without my having any chance to release them. An ocean of emotions trapped behind a face that looks like a mask—unchanging, motionless, and immutable. This is what I am: an expressionless figure that must work twice as hard compared to other people to communicate any mood. Sometimes this effort becomes three or four times as hard, and even more ... and it makes me so miserable, so frustrated, so tired.

So, Nancy, now you know what this is all about. You may think this is not that serious, and I would not blame you if you did. But this is *my* syndrome. This is *my* monster that I fight day after day, without ever being able to take a break.

This is *my* rarity. It has been my doom and my salvation, all in one.

The Sword in the Stone

There was a recurring phrase my parents used when I was a child: "You were unexpected." I never felt hurt, let alone offended by this statement. I knew they loved me immensely, and I never had any doubt about it. Quite simply, that phrase just meant that I arrived in this world at a time when my parents were not expecting to have more children. My mother, at thirty-six, was already heading towards a premature menopause. She would never have thought that the umpteenth missed period, similar to so many others, would mean pregnancy. She certainly was not ready for a surprise: she had already had a much more cumbersome one, twelve years earlier.

My parents lived a quiet life in a small village in Tuscany, in the province of Arezzo, near the medieval borough of Cortona. Located in central Italy, Tuscany is in many ways the heart of the nation, displaying in its territory the reminders of thousands of years of history. It had been the home of the Etruscans, whose elaborately painted gravesites litter the countryside. It had been the source of Italian language in the Middle Age thanks to such poets as Dante Alighieri, and it was the cradle of the Renaissance. We Tuscans are funny people. We love the arts and poetry, yet we are very practical-minded—a useful legacy of the past, given that the most powerful bankers of the Middle Ages resided in Florence.

My father was like that. Always an enterprising man, he was full of ideas and projects. He and my mother owned a grocery store, the only one in the village. It was more than enough for the small population—it would take *decades* before the first shopping malls appeared in the region—and it meant that everybody knew my family, and vice versa. Business was good but tough: seven days a week, no holidays, waking up early and going to bed late. Still, Dad yearned for more. He wanted his family to be financially secure, and he wanted a bright future for his offspring.

By the late fifties, Italy was gradually recovering after the tragic years of World War II, and was about to make a giant leap (the so-called Boom), turning from an agricultural-based economy to an industrial-based one. Industries were thriving, workers started moving from the countryside to the cities, roads and highways were being constructed as goods were being transported from one part of the country to the other, and cars—a rarity outside the big cities—were becoming more and more widespread. People had started looking to the future with confidence again after the ruin and hunger of the immediate postwar years. My father had sensed that things were changing and that the development of the road network and the growing use of cars meant new economic possibilities. Just as people needed food to gain energy, move, and work, so cars and trucks needed to be regularly fed—with fuel. Therefore, he opened a gas station just beside the grocery shop.

It was 1958, a few months after her wedding, when my mother discovered she was pregnant. There were no ultrasounds at that time, and in small country villages like the one where my parents lived, the common practice was to give birth at home, with only the help of midwives. Luckily, a doctor more diligent than others noticed that the baby's heartbeat was a little unusual, so he decided to have my mother hospitalized in the nearest town, just to be sure. There, after an X-ray, the only possible method in use in those days, the doctor's suspicions were confirmed: Mom was carrying twins.

The initial surprise over the number, which took everyone off guard, gave way to my father's annoyance when he discovered that, of the two babies, not even one was a boy. A dedicated football fan, Dad had bigger plans for his offspring. And so, the poor nun who came out of the delivery room, joyously announcing the happy event, had to face a bout of profane curses and swearing. We Tuscans are notorious for being hot-tempered and for using the name of God in vain, and my dad was no exception. That day he probably gave his very best. The new father of two beautiful and healthy babies, he had to abandon his plans for his son to become Italy's leading soccer player.

I always thought that having two sisters much older than I made me a very lucky little girl. Above all, I often benefitted from the fact that their characters were diametrically opposite: therefore, I could always count on each of them in a unique, special way, in different periods of my life. They were immensely different, yet at the same time they were united by an unbreakable bond.

Rossella, calm and thoughtful, spent most of her time with me in the years when I was just a happy little girl and not in the least aware of possessing the gift of *rarity*. She was the one who always came up with new games so that I wouldn't get bored and the one who looked after me when my parents were at work. She made everything look interesting and constantly stimulated my curiosity. She was a mother in miniature—sweet, careful, yet rigorous when needed. Rossella hardly ever got angry, but the few times it happened it was a sign that I had really done something awfully wrong. On those rare occasions, every word of reproach she said remained imprinted in my head and on my heart, indelible. I still remember the day I uttered my first four-letter word, most likely repeating what I had heard in kindergarten while playing with other kids: she turned very serious and told me categorically that never, ever again should I repeat a word so bad.

Later on, when I grew up, her advice was always clear. Measured, timely, accurate—even uncomfortable, sometimes, and decidedly not sentimental, but always correct and straight to the heart of the matter. To me, Rossella was like a rock, a cornerstone in my life. I knew she was there and that I would always find her when I needed her.

Tiziana, on the other hand, was outgoing and flamboyant, but she also had great sensitivity. I always felt comfortable talking with her about intimate things, the kind I would never tell anyone else—surely not Rossella, who was not so prone to sappy sentimentalism. Tiziana helped me a lot during my adolescence, when I was looking for so many answers to the problems in my life, when I felt lost and scared, when the entire world seemed to reject me. It was rewarding to talk with someone who sympathized totally with my mood, as a sister does. Only someone who has always been part of your life and who knows your insecurities, your fears, and your daily uphill struggle can understand certain feelings.

Tiziana was also very impetuous, sometimes arrogant. She never allowed anyone to overpower her, and for years I envied her assurance and her way of dealing with people. She was like a sword, capable of injuring, penetrating deeply, and yet extremely fragile, so much so that she would break if she came up against an obstacle just as tenacious.

In the family, we have always talked about them as "the sisters," as if they were unique in the world. And to me they really were. My first thought in the morning, as I woke up, was *Where are the sisters?* If they were away, even if it was just for a few hours, I asked, "When will the sisters be back?" If there was news of any kind, my main concern was, "Are we telling it to the sisters?" We used the plural, as if they were both doing the same thing at the same moment, always. Which says a lot about their symbiosis. As twins, they were so different from one another and yet complementary.

I remember when I was just a small child, we took a trip to the abbey of San Galgano, a beautiful and almost mystical ruined old church in the very heart of Tuscany. There, in the 12th century, a nobleman renounced his life of lust and violence to become a hermit after seeing a vision of the Archangel Michael. To symbolize his rejection of war and all things not sacred, the knight plunged his sword into the rock, which, according to the myth, "yielded like butter," leaving only the hilt exposed to form the shape of the cross. To some medieval historians, the story was held to be the origin of the myth of King Arthur. What I vividly remember from that trip was the sight of the sword, preserved and protected by a Plexiglas shrine. Years later, I found myself thinking that my two sisters were just like that—embedded into one another, inseparable—like a sword in a stone.

Perhaps because of the large age difference between us, "the sisters" always treated me like I was older than my years. Sometimes they took me with them when they went out with friends, and whenever that happened I was overcome with joy, since I felt like a "big" girl in their company. During the years when they attended teachers' training school, I was the perfect subject for the expression of their desire to become teachers: I was like a sponge that voraciously absorbed everything they taught me with so much love and dedication. Thanks to them, at just four years old I could read the simplest words, write my own name and count to one hundred.

The real teachers, in kindergarten, were always praising me to my parents, and my mother never missed an opportunity to tell everyone how clever and intelligent I was.

I was ashamed, of course. I wished that my mother would keep all that praise to herself, but even then I sensed it was her own way to highlight my inner gifts in an attempt to balance what I was missing from an aesthetic point of view. Less beauty but more intelligence, less charm but more friendliness. In thinking about it, my life has always been a long, grueling game of compensations—a game that had just started, and one I was destined to repeat over and over, like in a mad, never-ending replay.

Read My Lips

Going to kindergarten was quite a natural move, without any major trauma to it. I had the good fortune to live in a small town. I knew most of my peers and they knew me. None of them would ever dare to hurt me with cruel jokes about my appearance, because I was part of a community. True, I was a bit "special," but to none of them did I represent a *rarity*.

There was only one kid, decidedly exuberant, who kept spoiling my otherwise perfect days. He did not like me, not at all. However, the syndrome had nothing to do with that. Quite simply, I represented his total antithesis—his own personal nemesis.

I loved going to kindergarten. He hated it.

I was always receiving compliments from the teachers. He was constantly reproached.

At the end-of-year recital I played Little Red Riding Hood. He had to play the Big Bad Wolf.

And so, at the most unexpected moment, he would approach me from behind and kick me in the shins as if it were the most natural thing in the world to do.

"Ouch! You hurt me!"

"Who cares?"

"I'm telling teacher!"

"Who cares?"

"Then I'm telling my mom!"

"Who cares?"

The next day the same scene would be repeated, painful and just as frustrating. Soon my legs were covered in nice black spots and looked like a minefield. Meanwhile, my self-esteem (those days I had a good dose of it) began to waver.

As soon as she realized what was happening, my mother switched into total war mode. One day she showed up at the bus stop. As soon as my little tormenter arrived, I heard her utter these epic words: "The next time I see a bruise on my baby, I will come and slash your legs!"

Full stop. End of story. No more kicks in the shins. Justice had been done, albeit not in the most politically correct of ways. The rest of my kindergarten days were quiet and peaceful, whereas the poor boy's nights were probably haunted by horrible nightmares featuring the menacing leg-cutting witch.

And you know what? *Who cares!*

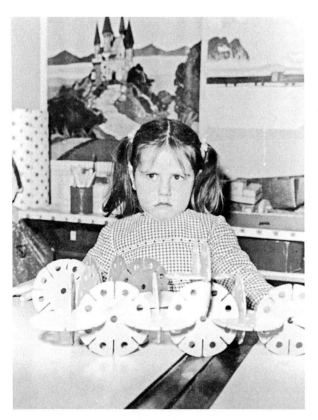

Winter 1974. At kindergarten, looking a bit intimidated because of the camera.

Instinct is a funny thing. Fascinating, if you think about it. Instinct helps us to not make mistakes. It stimulates our senses. Sometimes it can even save our life, although at first we don't realize it. Instinct had made me come up with a special way to talk, without my even being aware I had done so. I did not have functioning muscles around my lips; therefore, I was unable to pronounce those letters of the alphabet that required their use. Instinct made me find a shortcut. Whenever I had to pronounce a labial consonant—an "M," a "P" or a "B," instead of putting my lips together, which was impossible, I had my tongue come to the rescue. Pushing on the upper lip, the tongue replaced the lower lip, which refused to perform that function. It has always been like that, as far as I can recall. I don't remember when or how I found out that little trick. It's just been like that, always.

Now, I could not even conceive of a different way to speak—because, quite simply, there is no other way to speak, so far as I am concerned. Obviously, such a special method, such a personal system, has its limitations: some words sound a bit strange, distorted. A labial coming from my mouth does not have the crystalline sound it should, but most of the time people understand it all the same. However, since I am aware of not having perfect pronunciation, I am always ready to repeat a certain term twice or even three times, if necessary. That's the least I can do if I want other people to understand what I am trying to say.

I have always been very attentive to the listener's reaction, and I can guess right away if a particular word has escaped his grasp. No problem: let's just rewind the imaginary tape and repeat the phrase again, perhaps by changing some terms here and there in order to make its sense clearer and more comprehensible. It's a bit like when you are speaking in a foreign language and there are some words you don't know: you try to make do with a paraphrase, so as to express the same concept with terms you know better, even if it sounds a bit awkward at times.

What matters is the result: mutual comprehension. I really care about others "understanding" me, in all senses. I would like them to understand me despite my difference, and all that it implies. And if I do not start from that essential point—words—then I would have no hope of communicating. I could not reveal anything other than what is visible.

Since my early life was spent in the warm embrace of the small village community where I was born, everything went smoothly and without complications. No one paid any attention to my appearance or the rather "special" way I talked: they had known me since I was born and it was natural for everyone to accept me for who I was.

My awakening from this peaceful slumber began with the very first holiday of my life—or at least the first I remember consciously. Holidays had been a victory for my parents, a well-deserved luxury after years of hard work. My mother loved the sea, the sun, and the summer. I have never seen anyone enjoy sunbathing as much as she did. It was logical, therefore, that every summer our goal for the holidays was a seaside resort. Preferably it would be by the Adriatic coast, but anywhere would be fine, so long as there were sand, sun, saltwater—and a comfortable hotel where she would be "served and pampered," as she liked to put it, for at least a couple of weeks after her year of hard work.

So here we were, in Rimini, in one of the hundreds of hotels along the coast. I was five years old. The hotel was full of tourists, with lots of children of all ages and different nationalities. I had noticed that many of them were staring intently at me, only looking away after a long, obstinate overview. Still wrapped in my armor of innocence, I could not understand why they kept eyeing me in that way. Then, one evening, when he saw me coming, the tallest of the group pointed a chubby finger at me and asked me why I was *like that*.

"Me? What do you mean?"

Mean. "M." I had used my usual method, the one that came naturally, the old trick of the tongue pushed on the upper lip to pronounce the labial.

Big mistake. Only I didn't know that back then, and most of all I did not know of any other way to express those words. The kid started laughing in an exaggerated, obscene manner. And of course all the others followed him, without even knowing why—just wanting to join in the fun.

"Why do you talk like that?? You're weird!"

At that point there were two ways I could react. One: move forward towards my inquisitor, take that chubby finger in my hand and mercilessly twist it. Two: move backwards and run to the only warm and safe place I knew: my mother's arms.

I chose the latter.

Back in those days, there was in me not the slightest trace of bravado. Up to that time, there had never been the need to develop it. I was unprepared. The simplest thing to do, after being hurt so deeply, was to run away. And with that retreat came an end to at least part of my self-image as a beloved and hugged little girl.

A few days later, on the beach, another kid approached cautiously and asked my name.

"My name is Cristina."

Two "Ms" in one sentence. Damned labials. The kid looked at me a bit shocked and ran away as if he had just seen the Sandman, the Bogeyman and a werewolf, all at the same time.

By the end of that holiday, I was starting to put together a clear picture of my situation. And it didn't look too good. I was not a normal girl. Sometimes I aroused dismay, sometimes hilarity, and very often disgust. Not always, of course. Eventually, among the many children at the hotel, I had found a few of my own age who still liked to spend time with me. But more often than not it had been a constant banging against a brick wall.

Returning home I brought with me a new, sad awareness. I finally understood the meaning of the word *rarity*.

Pointed Fingers

In the months and years that followed, in elementary school, there would be many fingers pointed at me. There was always a new kid around, ready to raise his arm, stretch it outward, close the palm into a fist and let the forefinger spring out and diligently fulfill its task—that is, pointing at someone.

That someone was me. It was always, inevitably, me.

After some time, the pointed fingers started to look all alike, even though they belonged to different children, and those children became crueler and crueler. Each pointed finger was a reminder of how different I was, how abnormal. Each finger told me that I should be ashamed to be *like that*.

Oh, yes. Shame, shame, shame. And each time, after the finger came the question. Sure, it changed from time to time, but the meaning was always the same.

"Why do you talk *like that*?"

"Why do you laugh *like that*?"

"Why do you look *like that*?"

Like *what*?

Even nowadays, when I happen to meet some overly curious kid, I mentally play back the pointed finger scene as if in a movie, as if it all took place in slow motion. The little arm goes up and stretches out. Little fist. Little finger. And the question, which now I guess even before it is uttered because the meaning is still the same, even today.

But now I answer. Oh, do I answer.

Too bad I could not do it back then—nobody could. Not my parents nor my sisters, not my friends, and not even the doctors who had started studying my strange case. Nobody knew the answer.

It was frustrating, annoying, and especially painful. Whenever I ventured outside the idyllic community in which I lived, whenever I was travelling, whenever I was far from home, I turned into a more and more timid, fearful and shy little girl. Each pointed finger, each inevitable question had the effect of my taking one further metaphorical step backwards, further and further behind, more and more badly wounded. I wanted to hide, run away, become smaller and smaller until I would disappear. For a long, long time—preferably once and for good.

However, all was not lost. Just as in every fable worth that name, whenever I found myself in the most difficult situations I had my own personal knight ready to come and save me. Luca was a big kid; he was two years older than me. He was my second cousin, but to me he meant much, much more. We grew up together, lived a stone's throw away from each other, and of course I was mad about him.

Was he my best friend? No, more than that.

Was he my favorite playmate? No, no, much more.

He was my hero.

During the long stretches between lessons in the full-time school we both attended, he was always close to me and protected me from whoever tried to hurt me. He was my lifeline in that new environment, full of unknown children, some of them nice and friendly, others ready to unleash the most powerful weapon in the world: their pointed forefinger. Whenever this happened, my paladin came and stood in the middle between that powerful weapon and me. He was not particularly tall for his age, but to me he looked like a giant.

"If you keep annoying my cousin I'm gonna kick the hell out of you!"

Why had I to convey such violence all around me? Sure, it was a less splattery version of the leg-cutting witch evoked by my mother, but the result was just as effective. The little finger's owner suddenly turned into the fastest sprinter in the school—no, much more: the fastest in the whole universe.

Thanks to my protective cousin, my first years in elementary school were not experienced as a trauma. On the contrary, I loved going to school, I really did. Full-time was a perfect option: it was like living for half of the day within a second family. The teachers were nice and affectionate and represented lovable surrogates of my parents. My classmates—only ten children—soon turned into little brothers and sisters with whom I shared everything: study, meals, games—and the odd fight, just like in a real family.

We spent eight hours a day together, five days a week, and I never thought, not even once, that this place where I learned so many new and wonderful things was a tiring or unpleasant experience. At school I could express myself, my desire to stay with other people, my will to share experiences and feelings.

I loved every single moment spent with my new friends with all of my heart, and I had the distinct feeling of being generously reciprocated.

Behind the Mask

It was at that time, Nancy, that I began to understand the importance of communication. I learned quickly what it meant to "make up for" something. I knew I was lacking from a physical point of view. I would never be able to make people appreciate me because of my appearance, so it was necessary to find a solution, a replacement. I had to balance that gap with something that would be just as effective. Or at least I could try. It would not be easy, but I had to.

I just could not stand the idea of being rejected: that term was not included in my vocabulary. And I soon learned to my cost that to compete with such a powerful value as physical beauty was really complicated, an unequal battle if ever there was one, which almost always ended with the same result—defeat.

But I did not surrender. Time was on my side, and energy too. And a mind in continuous activity. You see, I always had to look for new ways to attract people's attention to my personality rather than to my outward appearance. To win that particular battle would become my main purpose in life.

I was starting at a disadvantage. The fact that I could not show my inner emotions through normal facial expressions was a big point against me. Each time I introduced myself to someone who had never seen me before, invariably my interlocutor would formulate the same thought and draw the same conclusion: no expression, no smile, no brain.

At first glance, for a split second, whoever saw me for the first time invariably wondered if there was a thinking mind behind that mask. I could tell this from their eyes. Taken aback, they just could not hide their thoughts. From that point onward, their reactions were different from time to time. Very different. After that first fraction of a second, most of them had already made up their minds about my state: I was incapable of reason. I was a mentally handicapped person. A subnormal.

Well, my friend, with that particular kind of person I just had no chance. I immediately gave up on any attempt at relating to them. And over the years I became pretty good at figuring out when it wasn't even worth trying.

Handshake.

"Hi!"

The smile turns off immediately. The hand withdraws a bit too quickly. The eyes convey the inference: she must be a mongoloid, at least. And maybe even contagious!

Good-bye. End of transmission.

From then on, the best reaction that I could expect from them was total indifference. From then on, I just did not exist anymore in their eyes, not even if I set myself on fire in the middle of the room. I was not part of any known species, therefore I could not exist.

Of course, not everyone reacted that way. Some were perplexed. The fraction of a second after the first impact, the one common to all—no expression/no brain—gave way to a shade of doubt on the face. The message was clear: they were offering me the chance to dissuade them from their wrong first impression. And it was that very moment when I had to give my very best. Those who offered me a second chance had the right to be rewarded.

Too bad a simple "hello" was not exactly the ideal way to express the best of me. There weren't many ways to greet someone; I could not prove that I possessed a brain by uttering a single word. So from that moment on began my painstaking work as an "enticer of souls."

I tried to come up with small phrases, possibly funny and interesting. I used a little trick that I invented at elementary school, with the teachers. I guessed the topic of the conversation and anticipated their next sentence. It might seem difficult, but actually all it took was a bit of concentration. You could always guess what they were aiming at. Therefore, most of the time I was ready to answer a question even before it was fully formulated.

That was quite an effective system. It always worked. It made me look more intelligent, more alert, smarter than average.

However, to entice teachers was too easy. I was playing a home game: school was the place where I had fewer difficulties in expressing myself. It was the rest of the world I still had trouble with.

But I would not give up that easily.

The Beginning of the Journey

And then it happened.

From one day to the next, my little world of stable and solid relationships was put in serious danger. When I was seven years old my parents decided to move to another, bigger house. It was only a few miles from the village I lived in, but to me it was as if I had been taken to the moon.

I was suddenly removed from my comfortable, safe nest and dragged into the middle of nowhere, in the countryside, where there was no one to play with. It could have resulted in a negative turning point, and yet, if I look back and go through the various stages in my life, I realize that in the most important phases my good star helped me. On that particular occasion, chance would have it that a little girl just one year younger than me lived in a farmhouse nearby. She literally saved me from the utmost loneliness, a condition I feared in a visceral way, then as now. Without my new friend I would not have known how to deal with such a radical change. I would have probably shut myself up like a clam, once and for all.

But no, I did not, thanks to Antonella. A quiet and sweet girl, the perfect playmate. I went to visit her with my mom the very day after we moved.

"Hi. I live down there. We just arrived yesterday. My dad says he'll build me a swing. A REAL one!"

From the huge smile that followed, I immediately knew we would become best friends. And so we did. We spent the whole day together during the summer holidays, always sharing the few toys that we had. The swing really made the difference: my dad always

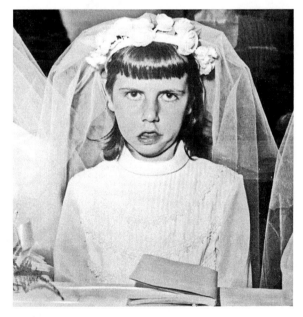

On the day of my first communion, 3 June 1978.

thought big and had built one made of iron, about 13 feet high, solid and unshakeable. We used to push each other harder and harder, and it never seemed enough. And we laughed, blissful in our conscious recklessness, in our graceful unconsciousness.

Antonella attended elementary school in a different village from the one where I was born, so we could not share that particular aspect of our lives, but for the rest we were inseparable. That was the time when I created the first real strong bond with another girl of my age. Antonella immediately accepted me for what I was, in a natural, disarming way. She never asked embarrassing questions, and she did not care about the strange way I spoke.

She had a little cousin, a few years younger than us. We had fun playing hide and seek and joining forces against the poor child, who went crazy trying to get the better of us in that or any other game. I guess you could call it girl power.

Antonella was my first real BFF. She would play a fundamental role, in the years to come, saving me from a very sad situation and introducing me to a new circle of friends. Once again, many years later, just as in our first encounter, she did not allow me to be overwhelmed by the condition that I have always feared the most—solitude.

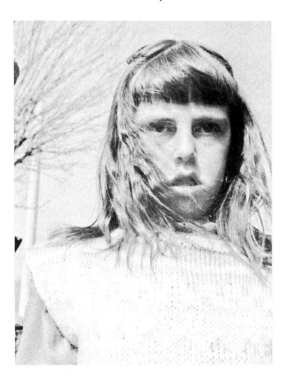

Winter 1978. A pic taken in my home garden. I was wearing a sweater done by my mom. Knitting for me was one of her passions.

However, my great love was school. Since we moved I had to use the school bus, which travelled beyond its normal route in order to come and collect me in front of my house. Fortunately, my parents did not consider the option of enrolling me in another institute because of that: such a decision would upset my habits and my way of relating with others. I was not ready yet to deal with an environment where I knew no one and that would probably turn out to be hostile.

Luckily my parents were aware of the trauma that they would cause making me change schools. They had immediately realized it would be a huge mistake. For my part, I was conscious of having been on the verge of a big crisis. Thank God I had not been thrown to the lions. This fact helped reinforce my deep bond with the school environment. Every time I crossed the threshold of my small class, it was like coming home. And every time I had to miss class I turned into a sad and disconsolate little girl.

I did not get ill often. My status as a "special" child did not affect in any way my overall health. In fact, my mom always told with pride that, of all the common diseases that affect children, I had only chicken pox. Oh, I remember it so well. Oh, yes, a period that more than made up for all the other childhood diseases I had so far escaped. However, if I had to miss school it was almost never because of my health.

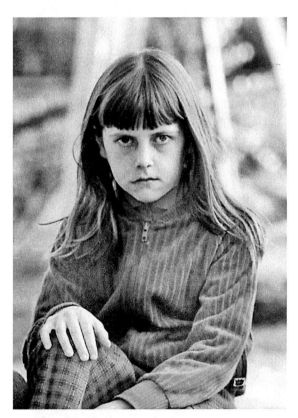

Until then, my parents had never investigated my condition deeply in search of answers or solutions to it. When I was still a very little girl, the simply did not have enough information to give to the physicians. But eventually I became big enough to answer the doctors' questions myself. After all, I was the one directly involved, and only I could describe

Winter 1979. I had long hair in that period, and dutifully posed for the camera like a little fashion model, my right hand posing on my leg as I had seen adults doing in magazines and films.

the problems that I had to face in everyday life, living side by side with the syndrome.

And so began our journey: an exhaustive search, a painful path that would lead us to understand the nature of my *rarity*.

Doctor Paolo and the Professor

You see, Nancy, there was another method that I often employed to catch other people's attention to show them I was a smart little girl, despite appearances. It was a variant of the anticipated answer. It consisted of concluding the sentence uttered by those who were addressing me, by guessing the right word and pronouncing it a moment before the person speaking did so. It is a trick I still use now and then.

To play in advance became a constant habit, like some kind of trademark. After practicing it for so long over the years, it has become so natural that sometimes I don't even notice when I'm doing it. Sometimes I probably exaggerate: it may sound pedantic, even priggish. But it is one of the best ways I have to let other people know that I am following their train of thought and I am right with them—even better, I am ahead. And it often works: all of a sudden I can glimpse a spark of interest lighting up in my interlocutor's eyes.

It's not love at first sight, mind you—I never expected that much. But at least this way I can dispel the hostility and mistrust that I have elicited in the first, critical moments.

It was this winning method that at the age of seven allowed me to captivate a new friend's sympathy.

Doctor Paolo was a young physician, just graduated in dentistry, and he was doing his internship in the hospital department where our search began.

"Hi, what's your..."

"My name is Cristina."

"Oh, well. Do you mind if I..."

"Ask me whatever you like. I'm here for this."

"Perfect. I really think you and me..."

"Of course doctor, we'll get along very well, I am confident of that!"

The mission now was, let's give a name to the syndrome. Actually, up until then we did not even suspect the existence of the word "syndrome." But it didn't stop there. We did not know anything—anything at all. My condition had simply been referred to as a "problem." No big words in my family, let alone at school. But now the time had come to find a more specific term, a definition to my—to our—"problem."

The odontology department at Perugia's hospital seemed the most logical place to start our journey. The city of Perugia was about one hour away from home: we could drive there and back several times a week if necessary.

Every visit there demanded a huge effort on my part. And it became increasingly onerous as the time and the months passed. I was seven and a trip to the hospital meant losing a day at school. I told you I loved going to school, Nancy, didn't I? What's more, it didn't take long to realize that it would not be easy to find the answers we were looking for. The road would be long and full of sacrifices. Month after month I was subjected to all kinds of medical tests, evermore strange, evermore annoying and invasive. And yet I felt a duty to support my parents in their attempts at figuring out what was wrong with me. They certainly didn't make those trips for themselves. They wanted to make my life better. They were moved by an immense love, and I would never stop them from showing it, in whatever way they chose. So I tried my best to behave. I was never naughty nor did I act up in any way. I never complained. I went to the hospital like a good girl and endured every kind of test.

Luckily there was Doctor Paolo. He made things so much easier to bear. His smile was warm and comforting and it was not easy to be indifferent to his kindness and sympathetic approach. Every time I had to undergo some further examination, he always made sure that everything was ready and in place so that I should not suffer any more than was strictly necessary. He was the first to meet me on my arrival and the last to greet me when I left, after yet another hard day of trial and error. I was gratified by his attentions, and of course I did not want to disappoint him. For this reason I tried not to complain or cry, even though the pain at times was unbearable.

With every visit there was some new test to face, and the names became more and more complicated.

Audiometry.

Ophthalmoscopy.

Encephalogram.

Cardiogram.

Electromyography.

My parents and I were taken through various departments, each time a different one, to check out every single part of my body. Not even the smallest detail would escape the examiners. And they engulfed us with questions that, in the end, all sounded the same. We answered their questions patiently but they never answered ours.

It was not easy to interpret the conflicting results that the doctors found through their tests. Sometimes they were astonished that a certain muscle worked when they thought it should not have. On the other hand, they could not explain why other muscles would not react as expected. So, just to be sure, they would check again.

And I found myself lying on a hospital bed, for the umpteenth time, waiting for someone to stick a thin needle into my flesh, between one muscle and the other, between one nerve and the other—in the face, the neck, the arms, everywhere.

It was not easy. Not even with Doctor Paolo telling me that there were still only a few minutes left at the end of each torture. Sometimes it was simply too much to bear: too much patience, too much resistance and too much pain.

Yet I never complained.

Sometimes I let fall a single silent teardrop, sometimes more than one. But that was all. I did not want them to think I was a capricious little girl, or that I was not cooperative. I wanted them to understand that I was really trying to do my best. I wanted to be accepted and appreciated. I was seven years old, and already I sensed that this was the ultimate goal. To be accepted. To be involved. To be part of them—the *normal* people.

The head of the odontology department, Dr. Paolo's supervisor, was a professor who followed my case with particular interest. I remember him as being huge, massive, awe-inspiring, and with a pronounced southern accent, something totally new and unique to me, which caused me intense discomfort whenever he spoke, rattling off one medical term after another. I felt intimidated, and I was not the only one. In his presence, no one ever dared speak unless spoken to first. When the "Professor" entered a room, no matter how noisy it was, he had the ability to reduce it to silence in three seconds flat. He was surrounded by an aura of tension that never left him. Every single word he spoke, in that strange unfamiliar cadence, sounded ominous, like a death sentence.

To me, he represented terror in its purest form. Then he turned into something else.

Usually it was Dr. Paolo who took care of my dental health. During each visit, he would check whether it was time to take out any baby teeth. On one of those occasions, the office door swung open without warning. It was the Professor.

The minute that followed his entry will remain forever in my memory as the most disconcerting that I ever lived through.

It all happened so quickly. After a fleeting glance inside my mouth, the Professor decided that one of my molars, a perfectly healthy one, should no longer stay where it was. It took him only two rapid movements to resolve the issue, without the slightest hesitation. The first movement was to take the pliers, the second to pull the tooth out with a force that seemed to me not even human—all this without anesthesia, of course. There was no time for that in the Professor's busy schedule.

The pain was devastating. No, it was explosive.

Even now, many years later, I can still see the disbelief on Dr. Paolo's face. He realized only that he would have to quickly dab the blood oozing from the open wound. Me, I thought I was about to pass out. Or maybe die, who knew?

Meanwhile, just as he had entered it, the Professor left the room in two quick strides. In the minute that it took him to extract my molar, he had not uttered a single word.

Well, thanks for stopping by, Professor. Come and see us again sometime.

Could Be Raining...

That morning we left early, very early, because we had a long trip ahead of us: almost 200 miles to get to Ancona in the Marche region. It was the nearest town I could undergo a rather new and still uncommon examination. Its full name was cryptic, intimidating, even alarming: computed axial tomography. What exactly was a "tomography"? What did "axial" mean? Why was it "computed"?

To reassure myself I tried to think about it by its abbreviation—CAT. That, I liked. It sounded much more familiar.

So here we were, my parents and I, in our small car, traveling through the Apennine Mountains. It was the longest trip I had ever made in my life so far and an adventurous one indeed. The Apennines are a fascinating mountainous region, and since it was mid-winter I could see the snow-covered peaks shining in the distance. Along the road, every now and then, a peasant stood near the road by his pickup truck, the trunk packed full with sacks of potatoes from his plot of land, a cardboard sign indicating the price per sack for whoever decided to stop and buy one. Then they disappeared behind us and we were alone, amidst the mountains.

Halfway there our car broke down. A few miles earlier it had started making weird noises, jolting and proceeding at an unsteady pace. Then it just stopped dead, in the middle of nowhere.

Mobile phones were science-fiction stuff in those days. My dad told Mom and me to stay in the car while he went to search for help. He showed up again after an hour with good news: he had found a bar with a public phone and called a mechanic, who would come as soon as possible with a new car at our disposal.

An hour passed. Then two. After three hours it became obvious that our savior had driven by without noticing us.

Despair.

What to do now?

We could only wait; there was no other option.

After another interminable hour of anguish, the mechanic finally showed up, arriving from the opposite direction from which we were expecting him.

Our delay was enormous. It took two more hours before we finally got to the hospital. Unfortunately our turn to use the CAT had passed, but we were told that if we had a little more patience, perhaps a remedy could be found.

Our patience lasted for four more hours of waiting but was eventually rewarded. I was incredibly tired when my turn finally arrived. They gave me an IV, which is necessary before the exam. Then I was placed inside a cylinder that reminded me eerily of a sarcophagus. I was warned not to move, not even an inch; otherwise I would have ruined everything, and we would have to repeat the test several times.

I was thirsty, unbearably thirsty. But I had to stand still, motionless.

And then there was the noise. Not a purr, but an ominous metallic rattle and clang which penetrated my ears and made me even uneasier. I would have plugged my ears with my hands if I could. Still, I could only wait, and wait, and wait—

I will remember forever those endless minutes, locked inside that torture instrument with the most bizarre name, which kept resonating in my brain like a mad tongue twister. A mixture of dread, anguish, and growing impatience, while the minutes dilated and seemed like hours.

Finally the torment ended and we were free to go home. Two hundred more miles from salvation. I still think of that day as the longest in my whole life.

Had I been born a few years later, I could have easily undergone the

CAT scan just a few miles from home. A few years later.... Sometimes this thought still crosses my mind, and I follow it and try to imagine *what would have happened if*... considering how many giant steps forward were made in medical treatment, technology, transportations.

Oh, well, never mind. To quote that classic Mel Brooks line of dialogue:

"Could be worse."

"How?"

"Could be raining."

Between one visit to the hospital and the other, time passed, and as my body grew up so did the problems. For example, when I clenched my teeth I could not close them completely: the doctors explained to me that such a peculiar character was named "open bite." The worrying thing about it was that the gap grew month after month, even though by just a few millimeters, and it was necessary to intervene immediately in order to try to halt the phenomenon.

We were told to go to a dental specialist who would create a customized tool suitable for my problem. Intervention was needed on two fronts: I needed to wear an appliance inside my mouth that flattened the palate and an exterior one I had to wear at night, which was designed to keep my bite closed while I was asleep.

I can't tell which I hated the most. It was really a toss-up. They were both small instruments of torture, each for different reasons.

The dental appliance was fixed. I could not remove it, and for months and months I was forced to speak with even greater difficulty than I already had. That hellish device did not allow me to use my tongue to speak as I was accustomed to, and the result was that little or nothing of what I was saying could be understood. Having to compete with yet another complication was humiliating. As if in normal life there weren't already enough of them. So, to avoid misunderstandings, I tried to keep speech to a minimum.

Perhaps it was in that period that a part of my character was shaped. From then on I never uttered a sentence if not extremely necessary, and I tried to avoid what was superfluous. Even today, I hardly launch into long monologues—save for this particular one, of course. I like simplicity, in general, but it is likely that all of this has to do with my proverbial laziness: since I don't like to make unnecessary gestures, I don't like to waste words.

I think I understood the true value of words in that period when I could afford very few. I had to weigh them, measure them and deliver them with difficulty only when absolutely necessary. I did not particularly suffer from that privation, as I was not a chatterbox, but what really disturbed me was that I could not give my best at school, during lessons, when the teachers questioned me. Naturally, they understood my objective difficulties, but it bothered me all the same not being able to express myself the way I wanted.

And that was only half the torture.

The other half stemmed from the device that I had to wear in bed—every night, for months and years. It was a chinstrap, which was supposed to sustain the chin during night hours, as during my sleep I was not able to control my jaw since I did not have enough muscles to do it. This strap was a set of elastic bands that wrapped around my head, crossed at right angles at various points and united under the chin, forcing my jaw to stay up and my bite to keep closed. Even too much, actually.

The doctor explained that the opening between the dental arches would still remain, but this way we would avoid its widening over the years.

Oh, sure. Message received, loud and clear.

Too bad that with that thing over my face I could hardly breathe at night.

Too bad that in the morning I woke up with a terrible pain at the base of my teeth and jaw.

Too bad the torment disappeared only a good hour after waking up.

The doctors tried to modify and perfect the damned device at every checkup, but each time the hassles were the same as before. In order to save me at least some of the pain, my mother stitched a cloth-and-cotton padding onto the lower part, around the chin, so that it would be less of an ordeal for me to wear it.

There was a saying that mom used to tell me in those years. *Chi bello vuol comparire qualche pena deve patire.* (Who wants to look beautiful must suffer some pain.) In Italian, it sounds sweet, like a caress, like a silly childish rhyme, and I suppose my mother knew it. She tried to defuse the situation and lighten the burden I had to carry; but I was not yet mature enough to take that saying in the right perspective. Beauty was a concept light-years away from me, and her words only served to feed my frustration.

And yet I never told her about that. I hurt her in many different ways, such as when I asked her why she brought me into this world, but I never blamed her for her good intentions.

Truth Revealed

Month after month, exam after exam, we were getting closer to our goal. Or at least it looked like that. We were about to give a name to my *rarity*.

The head of the dentistry department, the Professor—otherwise known to me as the Tooth Fairy after our unfortunate tête-à-tête—had been studying my case as best as he could and had collected the results of the many tests I had undergone over the years in a scientific and medical journal, *Rivista italiana di stomatologia* (Italian Journal of Stomatology) in the November 1982 issue. He was very proud to have discovered a case like mine, which he claimed was almost unique in the world.

Had he been provided with the technological means we have today, he would have soon noticed that I was not so special after all. However, in those years, the simple fact of assigning a name to a syndrome that had been scarcely known and studied was some kind of a record, to be kept in the utmost consideration. Furthermore, he had invested a lot in me— time, studies, and ruminations. The Professor's essay had a long and, to me, almost incomprehensible title: "Kinesiographic and electromyographic analysis of the masticatory muscles in Moebius Syndrome." However, those last two words stuck in my mind, where they would remain forever.

Moebius.

That was the name for which we had worked so hard, the name because of which I had suffered so much.

I started reading the article, which we had been kindly given free in a number of copies (you never know). It said this: "Moebius' syndrome is an extremely rare neurological disorder of which only 200 cases have ever been reported. It is characterized by bilateral paralysis of the facial nerves, usually nuclear, and is often associated with other cranial nerve (III, V, IX, X, XI, XIII) specific symptoms, as was the case we observed."

The *case* was me. And there I was, described in cold medical terms. It was a weird feeling, reading about myself as though it was a complete stranger, but one with the same characteristics, the same problems, the same deficiencies as me. Reading that article, I could see myself as the outer world was seeing me. And it was not a pleasant read. The article continued:

> The patient, a ten-year old girl, was affected by peripheral-type bilateral facial paralysis associated with partial paralysis of the trigeminal nerves. The lesions were present from birth, which was Caesarean section.... The

facies was typical and revealed the neuromuscular condition of her stoma-tologic apparatus. Due to the deficiencies of the facial and trigeminal nerves in the motor complex, all the muscles that depend on these cranial nerves were compromised. The forehead was flattened, the eyebrows inert; there was widening of the eyelid rims as a result of the paralysis in the lower lids and the patient had difficulty in both wrinkling her brows and closing her eyes. She, also, had difficulty in blowing and in pronouncing certain consonants, particularly labials. She could not masticate effectively and sometimes bit her tongue. Owing to the absence of blinking and the wide rims, foreign bodies often caused her eyes to water. When she used force to close her eyes the eyelids remained open but the eyeball rolled upwards (Bell phenomenon), whereas when she looked upwards the eyeball on the affected side rolled higher than the one on the healthy side (Negro phenomenon).

This case is particularly interesting from the point of view of the two cranial nerves that control the majority of the masticatory muscles and the consequent phonetic and aesthetic deficiencies.

The essay went on, illustrating the results of all the tests and measurements I had undergone in the previous months with all sorts of graphics and data. Among the "very interesting" results were these

The scarce muscular output in the mandibular kinetics had provoked hypoplasia of the condyles and marked widening of the mandibular angula-tion. This widening of the angulation and, naturally, the lack of muscle tone were responsible for the patient's inability to maintain a stable pos-ture, as well as for the exaggerated 10mm interocclusal free space.

Owing to the complexity of participation and muscle co-ordination, deg-lutination was extremely difficult for this child. The maxilla did not close adequately and in attempting to compensate for the scant retentive action of the orbicularis oris the child repeatedly placed her tongue between her teeth and pushed the saliva to the back of her mouth. Kinesiographic analysis, also, revealed other findings of interest. During mastication the myocentric occlusion varied continuously, so that after only a few move-ments the muscles already showed signs of fatigue and tremors started.

At this point the child was forced to help raise her mandible with her hands and to attempt to control the masticatory movements, the pathways of which were extremely erratic.

To illustrate these points, the article was accompanied by a series of pictures of this ten-year-old girl, the first a full-figure one taken on the beach—me with pigtails, attempting to smile at the camera. That pic must have been taken before the other kids started pointing their fingers at me. The following one had been taken at the hospital, while I was trying to perform those facial movements that, as described above, were severely compromised by my condition. One even showed my face caged in a weird mask-like apparatus next to a monitor—the kinesiograph. To an unaware distant observer, that weird little girl in pigtails was seemingly doing a series of grimaces, as in some sort of a silly little game. Perhaps, to that observer, those results were funny enough. To me, it was nothing short of heartbreaking. There I was, for all the world to see. That was me, and I could not hide from that awareness.

Now what? Now that we know all this, what's next for me, Professor?

"Oh well, first of all we will attend the next International Dental Conference and we will let everyone know what we have discovered."

Ah, well, sure, Professor. This will not help me, but it will definitely take you to the Olympus of the "rare disease discoverers." For you, all of this and more. After all, I have been your plaything for so many years that it would be unfair to deny you such a triumph—even though it will not bring any benefit to my situation or me. To diagnose a syndrome does not mean to cure it. And there is no cure for me, no solution to my problem.

But no matter, let's go to the conference and enjoy our fifteen minutes of fame. We did deserve them.

Those thoughts were never actually uttered. Too bad I was not yet brave enough: back then I was just a shy and scared little girl. Nowadays, I would say those words out loud; I would shout them at the top of my lungs. And then I would ask, "Did you hear me well, Professor?"

All I remember about that conference is the overall confusion: so many people wanted to examine me, observe me, and study me. At a certain point I burst out crying, and I don't even remember why. Too many emotions at once, perhaps. Or maybe too much undesired attention.

On the large screen in the congress hall a series of images were projected, with me as the sole protagonist.

Those were the pictures that had been taken of me over the years, during the many tests that I underwent, and watching them on a big screen was the worst part of the experience.

I never could stand to see myself as portrayed in pictures, and I still have some trouble tolerating mirrors. However, a reflection, an image, I can somehow change, I can relate. With pictures, there is nothing I can do: you are caught in that fraction of a second that takes the worst part of you and makes it immortal, and there is no going back. Not that I have much choice regarding the right timing: the chances of "looking good" in a pic are really scarce. So, Nancy, I definitely do not like pictures. I would go so far as to say I hate them. At the conference, those static poses, those shots amplified by the big screen, looked horrible, unbearable. In fact, everything was unbearable. And I could not wait to get away from those interested, inquisitive, hungry looks.

That day I even reassessed under a completely new light the insistent fixation of the finger-pointing children. At least, theirs was just ignorance—Father forgive them, for they don't know what they do. Whereas those doctors kept staring at me with a professional interest that I did not like at all. I perceived them as hostile, annoying and useless. None of them could ever help me by offering a magical solution. Therefore, it was time to go home and put my soul at rest. There was no way out. From then on, I would have to live with the Moebius Syndrome.

Forever and ever.

And so be it.

After that experience, my family and I were left with only two certainties.

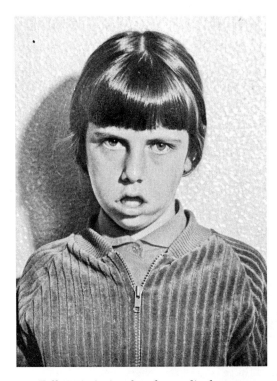

Fall 1979. A pic taken for medical purposes. It did not end up in the 1982 issue of the medical journal that examined my case, though.

One: the term "Moebius Syndrome" had been confirmed and approved by various experts.

Two: the only solution to my case would be a muscle transplant that unfortunately had not been perfected yet. Or perhaps a nerve transplant—or something like that. Very vague and not encouraging at all.

Meanwhile, as we waited for somebody somewhere to discover a way to move some muscle from one part of my body to another, the doctors had the brilliant idea to try to stimulate the muscles that were indeed in the right place but just wouldn't work. During each visit to the hospital, a new pastime awaited me: for at least an hour I was connected to a machine that sent

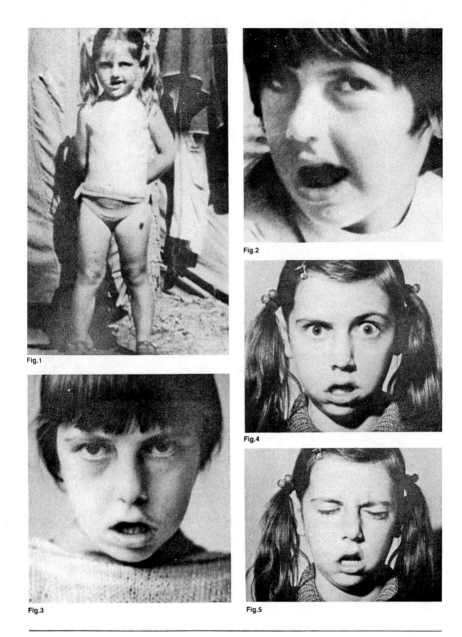

Fig.1

Fig.2

Fig.3

Fig.4

Fig.5

A page from the November 1982 issue of *Rivista italiana di stomatologia* (Italian Journal of Stomatology) which illustrated my case to the scientific community. There are five pictures of me. The first was one of my earlier pics, taken when I was five, at the beach, whereas the others were taken by the doctors in two different periods. I was asked to move my facial muscles and do various grimaces for the camera (courtesy ANDI).

electrical impulses to sensors applied on my cheeks, on my forehead, near my eyes. Mild electric shocks, just to add a little bit of "spark" to my situation.

For the first half-hour it was tolerable, then it turned into a torment. I had to invent all kinds of mental games to pass the time, as an electric

Rivista Italiana di Stomatologia 11/82

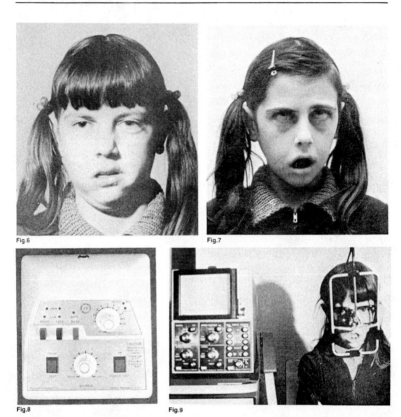

Fig.6   Fig.7

Fig.8   Fig.9

e a determinare la relativa posizione di riposo alla luce della moderna teoria neuromuscolare di B. Jankelson (1, 2, 3).
Secondo tale teoria la posizione di riposo viene intesa come quella posizione della mandibola nella quale i muscoli sopra-ioidei e sot-

reproducibility is unobtainable in the same subject with the myomonitor and the mandibular kinesiograph (4, 5, 6), the value of the rest position is obvious. The myomonitor (Fig. 8) is a galvanic stimulator which trasmits electrical impulses to the Vth and VIIth nerve

Another page from the medical journal, with two pics which illustrate my difficulty in closing eyelids and the eyeballs anomaly related to it. The pic on the lower right half illustrates the device for the electrical stimulation of the facial muscles I had to wear during the sessions (courtesy ANDI).

shock punctuated each and every second. Luckily I did not lack imagination, or patience. And I needed both in massive doses during those sessions.

It went on like this for a few months, and finally, given the almost zero results, the Professor decided it was time to stop.

Rivista Italiana di Stomatologia 11/82

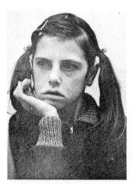
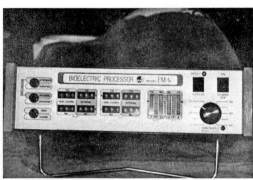

Fig.28   Fig.29

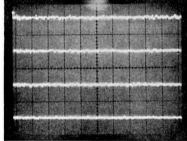
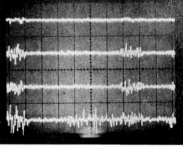

Fig.30   Fig.31

ta allora come durante la sua esecuzione le mascelle non vengano adeguatamente serrate, ma anzi come fra i denti venga ripetutamente interposta la lingua nei tentativi ripetuti di vicariare la scarsa azione ritentiva dell'orbicolare della bocca e di spingere la saliva verso il retrobocca (Figg. 25-26).
L'analisi kinesiografica ci consente ancora altre considerazioni. Durante la masticazione si evidenzia come la occlusione miocentrica varia continuamente e come dopo pochi atti i

was scarse both at resting (Fig. 30) and under force (Fig. 31).

Conclusions

In analyzing this rare clinical case we have tried to demonstrate the lack of a rest position and to show that this is the result of a muscular equilibrium which, in the present case, was extremely deficient. Furthermore, electromyography and mandibular kinesio-

An electromyograph with surface electrodes was used to monitor the electric activity of my muscle. The top left pic illustrates my habit of helping raise my mandible with my hands during mastication (courtesy ANDI).

"Thanks everybody for allowing us to try. If we hadn't tried we wouldn't know, would we?"

No. I *did* know.

But I don't think he would have listened.

Laura—Part One

Each time, after those grueling sessions, coming home was like being born to a new life. If anything else, I had the opportunity to appreciate the difference between a quiet life and one characterized by the submission to instruments of subtle torture. As long as you don't experience pain up close, you are never aware of how lucky you are when you don't have to fight it. I discovered this very soon, thanks to the shock-spitting machinery.

However, as my sister Rossella would say, you should always look on the bright side of things: thanks to those unpleasant and annoying experiences I could better enjoy the happy moments, far from the hospital, in a much deeper way. I savored them in complete, utter absorption. That's why, looking back, I can say I had a happy childhood. In spite of everything, I was a serene little girl.

Then, like everyone else, I started to grow up, leaving behind the naivety of childhood. By middle school, the situation had evolved, and my needs and priorities had changed. A stubborn, obstinate temper was starting to emerge, and it would help me in the following years to fight my way in life. I wanted to excel in everything I did, and to compensate for physical deficiencies, as I had done in the past, I kept trying to display my hidden inner qualities, which otherwise no one would have noticed. And I would have easily succeeded in getting the best out of all my young classmates, if it were not for her.

Laura.

We had known each other a long time, having attended the same schools since kindergarten. She was born exactly six months before me, in late spring, while I came to life in late autumn. This very detail always struck my imagination deeply: it was as if this fact put us at the opposite sides of an imaginary line—a perfect metaphor to describe our eternal love-hate relationship.

She was cheerful, bright, and naturally beautiful. I was shy, introverted and hopelessly ugly.

And yet our enormous diversity somehow united us. Whenever we were not engaged in trying to prevail over one another, we realized that our friendship was stronger than anything else. The problem was that, from an early age, we both were extremely competitive. Each classroom test, each interview became a battle of vital importance that had to be won at all costs, by any means. And often I did win—but school started losing the importance it had in the past years, and thus my victories were losing much of their meaning.

In those years I started to discover that another, much more fascinating world existed, and one that affected my adolescent imagination much, much more: the male universe.

And in that field I was no match for Laura.

Her magnetic charm, her crystalline laughter, her exquisite grace could make anyone fall at her feet. And of course, the first to surrender were the boys who should have been interested in me, in my little teenage dreams. And yet, not only I was not even deigned a look, I also had to resign myself to the idea that Laura would be the focus of each and every one of those looks, the kind that I desired so intensely.

It was not right.

Oh, no, no, no and no.

In our first school trip, students from a nearby village joined us. It was a new and exciting situation: we would meet boys we had never seen before. And of course I fell in love. Madly.

He was tall, blond, with beautiful blue eyes and the quaint charm of the "stranger." However, the chances of a tender love story blossoming between us amounted to zero, and I was well aware of it. Still, this did not stop me from filling page after page of my school diary with colored hearts and sappy lines taken from who-knows-what Z-level romance novel. In chronological order, day after day, written with a silver marker—a novelty in the early eighties—one could read the following assertions:

> Up with me, Cri Cri
> Up with Cristina
> Up with me and ... Him
> Who will be my Prince Charming?
> Up with l'amour (what a poetess!)
> Up with health
> Up with intelligence
> Up with family
> Up with technical education
> Up with math
> And after so many "Up withs" we need some "Down withs"

Down with illnesses
Down with sadness
Down with melancholy
Down with Laura.

The diary was dedicated to the cartoon character Candy Candy, the heroine in the anime television series of the same name—my favorite. Of course, in my own fanciful psychodrama, I played Candy while Laura perfectly embodied Eliza Leagan, the whimsical, haughty, aristocratic girl who constantly insults and humiliates Candy. Indeed, she even looked like her! And, like Eliza, she was always trying to put a spoke in the wheel. If I wasn't careful, she would take everything from me. Not just the boys, but also my friends.

"Even if Stefania's best friend will be Laura I won't take it personally and Stefania will also be my best friend, whereas I hate Laura because she attempts (and succeeds) to steal her from me."

The reasoning was flawless—except perhaps from a grammatical point of view.

"Laura's flaws: uncaring, deceitful, spiteful, malignant, *arfacimosa*, thief."

Apparently a puzzling neologism, to me *arfacimosa* (a term that does not exist in the Italian vocabulary) could actually be attributed to many characters—all of them execrable.

Beautiful and well aware of it (bad). Presumptuous and walking a good two feet off the ground (very bad). Self-centered, always craving everybody's attention (very, very bad). Vain, boastful, haughty, arrogant, selfish (the devil incarnate).

The only weapon I had left was academic performance, which was often more favorable to me. Those were fleeting victories, which, however, renewed after every classroom test, allowing for brief jubilation.

Then, when the pages of my beloved Candy Candy diary began to look too crammed to keep all my original and brilliant thoughts, since the school year had rigid time limits, at the age of thirteen I allowed myself the luxury of a secret diary.

Hardcover, solid, of substantial weight, decorated with a pink stripe on the left side and many, many colored hearts in the middle. Most important thing of all, it had a steel padlock.

Inviolable.

The key, the only instrument that could open that lock, was always with me. I kept it concealed in my pocket. Better be careful. Mine were important secrets, better not risking.

Dear Diary,

Today is the first time I write on these pages and I'm quite excited because I've never kept a diary. I just wanted to tell you that I'll be thinking of you as a true friend in the flesh because I've never had any. You know, I purchased you over a month ago, but since I like special days I waited for one to start writing on your pages: in fact, today I am precisely thirteen years and six months old.

Today is also the birthday of a friend who's called Laura, but to tell the truth she and I were born to hate each other and be rivals in everything.

Better be clear right from the start. No doubt from the very first lines, dedicated to my own personal nemesis.

Dear Secret Agent,

First of all I want to apologize because it's been a long time since I last wrote. Then let me inform you that on June 30th I finally knew the results of middle school's final exams and I am happy to announce to you that I got an A, whereas Laura got an A-! You can imagine my joy, as I finally got the better of my greatest rival.

Take that. The victory of victories. And from then on, it was downhill all the way.

We both chose, the only ones in our school who did, to attend the classical lyceum in Cortona, the medieval town on the hill that dominated the surrounding area. It was a wonderful feeling, every morning, travelling along the curvy road that led to the top of the hill. Looking down from the bus, we could see the whole valley and, far in the distance, the lake Trasimeno—a breathtaking view, as was the sight of the huge angular stones that formed the town walls dating back to the Etruscans. And then there were the narrow alleys, the churches, and the town hall and its imposing stone stairway towering over the main square. It was almost too beautiful to bear, and it made my love for school even stronger.

In the first months of lessons, I minutely recorded in my diary every mark I was given, so as to emphasize each time I managed to overcome Laura in class assignments and oral tests. Then, incredibly, one day I wrote this:

Dear Diary,

On the 12th we had our Latin test and the professor brought it back yesterday: I got (and please do not faint!) A+! Whereas Laura just got a C-. What a shame! She got a lesser grade than most in the class. Now she doesn't bother me anymore, and instead of hating her I'd like her to be given much better marks—it being understood, not as good as mine.

Generous, but without exaggerating—*it being understood.*

And yet, without even realizing it, I adored her. Laura was my alter ego, the person I wanted to be—not just because of her physical appearance, which I envied immensely, but especially for her charisma, the ability to attract people in a natural, instinctive way. She was an inspiration on a myriad of occasions. She advised me on how to dress, which hairstyle to choose, what kind of music to listen to. And I followed her suggestions to the letter: they always seemed to be right, in each and every field.

My wardrobe underwent a revolution, with the inclusion of miniskirts, trendy denim jeans and pointed boots. I started going to the same hairdresser as Laura and one day I came out with a brand new perm which looked totally eighties, but I absolutely loved it. After all, hey, those *were* the eighties!

Of course Laura had beautiful and natural curls of her own—who could doubt that? To console me, she always told me that she envied my nondescript straight hair, uncooked-spaghetti style. I was so lucky to have it! Nice try, Laura, but I never believed it. At least, now we had one thing in common. Or should I say one *more* thing in common? You see, I was working on other fronts.

Regarding music, for instance, I had debatable tastes to say the least. Sappy Italian melodic singers, trendy British new romantic bands, one-hit wonders that would be forgotten within a few months. Laura's bedroom, on the other hand, was a marvelous world where I used to get lost for hours and hours. She lived in an old country farmhouse, a typically Tuscan style, built of stone and with thick inner walls covered with a layer of rough plaster. In Laura's room the walls were crammed with hand-made writings: reflections, thoughts and famous quotes. Each time I paid her a visit I found some new ones, squeezed into some of the few empty spots. And then there were the posters: The Doors, Led Zeppelin, The Cure, and an Italian punk band I had never even heard of: CCCP. Thanks to Laura, my musical training was saved and irrevocably diverted to much healthier directions: she gave me cassettes on which she had taped her favorite records, and each time she fell for a new band or artist she made me part of her discovery—to my utmost joy and gratitude.

We started ganging up at small concert venues, and it was lots of fun getting in touch with those new, unknown environments. There, no one looked at me in a strange way: everybody seemed to be minding their own business, listening to good music and jumping in time with it. Which was exactly what we did too: I, Laura and her younger brother, whom I suspected had a certain influence on his sister's musical tastes. Somebody must have given her tips, after all—it couldn't have been just her own work!

Laura's brother had a troubled past behind him. He was no less than the evil little kid who had fun kicking my shins at kindergarten, the one whose legs my mom threatened to cut off, the one who for a long, long stretch must have avoided the phrase "Who cares."

Who knows—perhaps he eventually discharged his violent childhood tendencies into a cathartic abandon to rock music. It amused me to think it went like that.

First Love

Dear Little Secret Agent,

Yesterday, during the test, Laura asked Ferdy for help and he, silly as he is, tried to gave her tips while the professor was outside for a minute, telling us to come back inside: as soon as we finish the test, we walk out of the classroom so as not to disturb the others. In short, the professor caught Ferdy in the act and gave him a lower mark as a punishment. I felt very sorry for him, because I kind of like him, but of course the feeling is not reciprocated.

Ferdy—short for Ferdinando—had been my desk-mate since the very first day in high school. That's how we met. By sheer chance we happened to be placed next to each other, just one of so many chances. Always the passionate fatalist dreamer (which I am still today), I interpreted it as a sign of fate. However, it was not a typical case of love at first sight—but something very close.

It took me just a few days to figure out he would be the ideal desk-mate: nice, kind, funny and, above all, sensitive, competent and clever. I had just met a new competitor.

Once I had absorbed the idea that the eternal struggle with Laura was by now unequal, I had turned my attention to somebody else—one who often gave me a hard time. And occasionally he even got better marks than mine.

That cheeky fellow! How dare he?

I just had to put the record straight and show him he would not have an easy time. And, most of all, I had to play all my cards to try and win him with my charm. Because, despite the hassle of being outdone at school, I just could not be angry with him. As a matter of fact, I liked him. I liked him a lot.

He had a sense of humor very similar to mine, so much so that during lessons we used to chatter softly and giggle all the time. I knew I had to restrain myself: it never occurred to me to be reproached that often by the professors, but I could not help it. Every opportunity we had to exchange views, feelings, and jokes was a shock to my heart.

As if by magic, the name Ferdinando began to appear in my secret diary more and more often. The endless list of marks obtained in class assignments and tests was now totally devoted to the competition between Ferdy and me, which had decidedly ousted the historic but now emotionally empty one with Laura.

The clash between Ferdy and me in educational achievements was my pathetic attempt to get as close as possible to Ferdinando's heart. I was hoping that by keeping up with him, and trying to get better marks than he did, one day he would finally notice me, appreciate me, even love me. Still, I had no illusions. Despite my daily dreams, I was a rather realistic type after all. I could never pretend that he loved me. I would settle for less, much less. I would have been more than happy if one day he would address me with just a miserable, pathetic "I am fond of you." And that day came. There were no official statements, nothing explicit—God forbid. However, to me it was important all the same. I would never erase that day from my memory, ever ... at least for the following years in high school. And perhaps a little more.

We went on a school trip to visit Rome, on a beautiful spring day. It was my first time in such a big city, and the majesty of its monuments impressed me a lot. However, that day—in spite of all the natural and historical beauty we admired—another thing proved as indelible in my heart: the journey back home.

Dear Diary,

Today I found out that Ferdy got a C in the Latin oral test, which I still have to undergo, which worries me a lot. However, let's move to the most exciting thing of the day: the trip to Rome. As a school trip, it was routine, I'd say: we visited the Trevi Fountain, the Coliseum and a very boring museum. I liked Rome a lot—I didn't expect it to be *that* huge.

But the most important thing happened during the trip back home. I was sitting next to Ferdy, and up to now it was almost normal as there were five of us sitting in the back of the bus. At one point our classmate Stefania joined us and started teasing Ferdy, tapping him gently, hugging him and flirting all the time. Then she leaned her head on Ferdy's shoulder and I don't know why, but I did the same. And that alone was a very exciting occurrence. Even though he kept playing silly with Stefania, I kept telling myself that I loved him and my love grew more and more, minute after minute.

But the best was yet to come. Laura wasn't sitting near to us, so Stefy started talking about her, saying things that I've been repeating since I know Laura—that is, she is a great opportunist, she becomes friends with some other girl only when she needs something from her, and when she does not need that person anymore she tells her to go to hell. Stefy was amazed and disgusted because she would never have expected that. At first I didn't pay much attention to her words, as many other people said the same about Laura but later on things turned out the same as before. But Ferdy agreed with her and I intervened too, telling that Laura had her own way with boys too. Ferdy replied that he knew it perfectly well. I was amazed, and told him I did not believe him, because he had fallen into her trap as well. But Ferdy told me he would never make that mistake again, and that he knew that Laura was just coaxing him into letting her copy his homework and things like that. You can't imagine the joy I felt when I realized that he was well aware of that! I tried to warn him by telling him that sooner or later he would be falling back into her trap, but he assured me otherwise.

In fact, it was a very confidential moment: he told me some things I did not know and I did the same. In the depths of my heart I hope that he will never forget this evening—I surely never will. It was the first time I spoke that frankly with him—or any other guy, for that matter. I told him that I was not interested in him, but I was sorry to see poor boys like him "wasted" that way. And he smiled at the word "wasted." I repeated that I was not interested in him personally, because I am afraid that he should find out how much I do like him ... even though I think that maybe, VERY VAGUELY, he noticed it.

Well, it's kind of late now and I must say goodbye, but I want you to know that even though this seems a very little thing, it made me immensely happy because now I know Ferdinando listens to my opinions and appreciates me *for what I am.*

That day three things had happened which had upset my whole life deeply.

The first was that I had a physical contact—imperceptible, yes, but provoked by me—with a member of the opposite sex. Leaning my head on Ferdinando's shoulder—or that of any other boy on the planet—was a new event, something risky and unthinkable at the same time. Until that moment I had carefully avoided touching or even being very close to anyone I hadn't known for at least a decade—which meant a lifetime, more or less.

Over the years, I had become aware of the discomfort I caused in other people, whatever gender or age they were. As an adolescent, that belief had become rooted in me permanently, especially in connection with my peers: I avoided any verbal approach if I sensed it was not welcome, and I always realized it in a matter of seconds. To approach someone for a physical contact was out of question. Among other things, I always had the feeling that many of those who were looking at me in a strange way were probably asking themselves whether mine was a contagious disease. Best to avoid any contact, then. Best for them, and even better for me.

Instead, in that magical journey back home, I had gathered all the courage I could and ventured into an attempt at a physical approach. And Ferdinando did not move back, nor did he show any sign of annoyance. He did not hurt me in any way. The fact that he was busy flirting with my classmate, and acting a little silly, was just a superfluous detail.

After my glorious first victory in battle, I now firmly believed I had supernatural powers and was convinced that if only I thought very intensely, with all of my will, that I loved him, I would transmit a good amount of that pure feeling to him. It had to work like that: the one person who had not rejected me would surely perceive my feelings for him as well, since he was gifted with such a massive dose of sensitivity. No doubt about it.

The second cause of excitement was the fact that someone finally realized what I had been arguing for a lifetime: the theory that I carried on tenaciously for years and years had been enunciated aloud by another classmate. And not only that, it had been confirmed as well, by the person I cared about the most: Ferdinando. Laura, my eternal rival, had been unmasked, and finally truth would win over all.

What satisfaction! The proper reward after so much effort on my part. I couldn't believe it. Surely it would be a short-lived victory, because no one could escape the undisputed charm of the temptress par excellence. Therefore, I exhorted others to pay attention to what awaited them. Laura the seducer was always lurking, a constant danger. In the meantime, that night I was savoring the taste of complicity that I had reached with my new flame. It took very little to make me happy, after all.

Last, something happened that I did not dare hope for. Ferdinando opened his heart to me. He told me "some things" and I did the same. We reached an intimacy that I had never experienced before, with any guy in the world. Small talk had become the open door to God-knows-what future prospects, and that thing made me euphoric.

O dreams, come to me.

O hopes, gather from everywhere.

Here history is being made, but let nobody notice, please.

No one has to know—or at least, only *very vaguely*.

Laura—Part Two

Laura, her brother and I spent all the holidays of my adolescence together. Since our mothers were best friends, being a few weeks together each summer on the Adriatic coast had become a fixture none of us would give up. We grew up sharing the same experiences and common spaces. The only difference was that Laura's spaces were always full of people and mine were not. Despite of all her efforts to introduce me to her new circles of friends, there was not much to do. I was usually not accepted as an interesting presence.

Laura had the gift of becoming friends with everyone mere minutes after the first encounter, whereas I needed days just to have the honor of receiving regard worthy of this name. And I was pretty sure that most of the times such regard, even though minimal, came from the fact that she wouldn't make one step without me. The one condition for being allowed to enjoy her company was to have me included in the package as well. All or nothing.

I was acutely aware that without her my summers would have been anonymous and insignificant, whereas my holidays with Laura all had a unique flavor, a vital energy worthy of our adolescent age. We used to go out every night, and every time with new and different friends; we went to discos, pubs and clubs, and dived into the crowd until the early dawn.

We lived as in a train moving at supersonic speed, and most of the time I was glad to be a passenger in that particular compartment. Better be part of it than watch it pass by without being able to get aboard.

Even though the velocity was too high for me.

Even though sometimes I would want to slow down and leave.

But I was aware that if I hadn't moved at that velocity—*their* velocity—there would have been one and only one alternative. Isolation. This was a perspective so terrifying that it could not, it should not, be taken into consideration. And so, as my favorite superhero used to say, "Up, up, and away, faster than the speed of light!"

That very same energy I accumulated during the summer period should have been sufficient for the rest of the year, back from the holidays, according to Laura. But as I got home again I went back to being the shy and awkward girl who felt at ease only within domestic walls, because I knew that outside there was no big news awaiting, neither at school nor elsewhere.

Still, Laura did not give up.

In class, during lessons, she kept sending notes.

Tomorrow night at the disco, are you coming?

I hated discos. I hated that noise that would not allow you to listen or be listened to. For somebody like me, with a desperate need to communicate with others, they were hellish places where any attempt at mutual conversation would burn out. Besides moving in an unnatural way, I could not do anything else. And with all that noise, I certainly could not express my inner self. In a disco, nobody could care less about my inner self.

No Laura, I don't feel like it.

I gave the note back to my desk-mate, and the little piece of paper was passed from hand to hand until it reached its original drafter. Then, a few minutes later, it returned to me.

Come on Cri, we'll have fun, I swear!

How insistent. Phew, unlikable. How could she not understand?

No, I don't feel like it, I'll just be bored. Too noisy.

Another passing of the baton, and back.

Cri, if you're not coming I won't go either. You wouldn't want to tease me, right?

Guilt. How could I disappoint her? No, I certainly couldn't.

Ok, but we'll be back early, ok? There's a classroom test the day after tomorrow.

Note leaving, note coming back.

Deal! You'll see; we'll have fun! Thanks!

Thanks. For what? It was she who was doing me a favor. It was one of the hundreds of attempts to make me share a part of her life. I was perfectly aware of it and loved Laura for that, even though it always cost me much to give up to her little blackmails for a good cause—because in the end I never had fun like she promised I would.

It was not Laura's fault, of course: other than drawing me into her world, there was not much that she could do. The rest of the job I had to do by myself.

If only I had been the smooth-talking type. But I was locked in myself, insecure and practical at the same time. I loved essential phrases—no frills or nonsense—whereas social life in those years was a matter of superficial, trivial conversations.

And yet I would not bend to the common rules of *savoir vivre*. Talking about banalities bore me to death. Yet the main topics that everyone talked about were all the same, and there was no way out. School, boys, homework, boys, holidays, lipstick, cigarettes, boys.

The Fifth Canto

"Now, boys, today we're going to have an oral test on Dante's *Divine Comedy*. Let's see who is going to be the chosen one this time."

Absolute silence in the classroom. Static energy, and a palpable tension can be read on everyone's faces. The class register opens, and the professor's finger scrolls over the names. Up and down, and then up and down again.

"Let's see ... uhm..."

Anguish, faster heartbeats, sixteen young students holding their breath and all thinking the same thing. Please, please, please, move that finger away from my name. And like everybody else, in this moment I am focusing all my mind energy in trying to keep that finger away from mine.

"Let's call ... let's call..."

Eyes lowered on the books in the hope of being able to camouflage— or rather, to disappear—sucked into them as if by magic.

"Well, let's.... On second thought, today we'll toss up a number."

Panic.

I wonder if anyone wrote a book on the subject, something like *A Hundred Ways to Torture a Student*. Tossing up a number means that the professor is going to choose a number and then call the corresponding name in the class register, according to the alphabetical order. Me, I am Number Four.

To pick the number, the professor opens a page of the book at random. Now it's all a matter of fate, and mathematics.

"Sixty-seven. Six and seven makes thirteen. Sciarri Lorena."

Who said thirteen was not a lucky number? Poor Lorena, pity it was her turn, but better her than...

"Oh, no, too bad, Sciarri is absent today. So, did we say thirteen? Well, then let's make it one plus three. Which makes four."

Fifteen sighs of relief, fifteen silent "Thank yous" addressed to heaven, fifteen cardiac muscles back to a normal rhythm. But not mine.

I knew it had to be me, just the one day that I didn't study properly. Murphy's law, they call it.

I get up and head towards the teaching post with the look of a prisoner advancing along death row. On the way to the blackboard I mentally summarize the previous lessons: the whole of Italian literature in ten seconds flat. Maybe fifteen. But it only makes me more and more upset.

When I stop by the teaching post, I am fully convinced that this is going to be a disaster waiting to happen, but I have to show some self-assuredness. I cannot let my utter bewilderment transpire.

Sometimes, lacking a functioning facial mimicry can be quite useful.

"So, Cristina, let's talk about Dante's *Inferno*—the Fifth canto."

Three hypotheses come to my mind

Inferno. Hell. That's where I am right now. What a sad irony and easy to describe. A mixture of sorrow, inquietude and negative thoughts.

Inferno. That's where I am going for not having studied enough—and rightly so. I fully deserve it.

Inferno. *The Divine Comedy*. Fifth canto. "There Minos stands, hideous and growling, / Examining the sins of each newcomer: / With coiling tail he judges and dispatches." The sad love story of Paolo and Francesca. They are placed in the Second Circle, where sins of lust are punished. Among the souls are Cleopatra, Helen of Troy and Achilles. "Francesca, your sufferings / Move my heart to tears of grief and pity. / But tell me, in the season of sweet sighs, / By what signs did love grant to you the favor / Of recognizing your mistrustful longings?" Francesca speaks, while Paolo stays silent and cries. Dante is so overwhelmed by pity that he faints. "And I fell just as a dead body falls."

I know it! I know everything about the Fifth canto! I can do it! I definitely can!

"In the Fifth canto of Dante's *Inferno*, Dante and Virgil reach the Second Circle and meet Minos, who..."

A hesitation. What was that? I felt like something just ripped inside my face.

"They meet Minosse who has the function of..."

Ouch! Again, and now it was much more painful. What's happening to me now?

"...the function of judging the souls of the damned..."

Damn it. Now I can no longer speak. The words I am uttering come out unintelligibly. My jaw is imperceptibly twitching and moving sideways—*by itself*. I stay stunned for a split second, and then I try to react. I try to push it towards the opposite direction with my force of will.

At first I succeed because the twitching is slight. But as soon as I relax my muscles, the jaw returns to its unnatural position and keeps twitching. And now it hurts, it really hurts. I have to use my hand to put it back in place, pushing hard.

What is happening to me? I never, ever experienced such a thing before. It is as if my jaw has a life of its own.

All of a sudden, I realize the teacher is watching me, looking quite worried. I must be an interesting phenomenon, seen from the outside. A flow of blood rushes to my face. I feel ridiculous, standing there before the teaching post, with one hand trying to hold back a part of my body that suddenly seems to have gone mad.

All eyes are on me. And I'm in pain. *In pain.*

What if it never comes back in its place? What if my jaw stays like that, dislocated, in an unnatural position for the rest of my life? Can I endure this? Can I tolerate the pain? And then what? What more? What will be next?

I do not have the time to answer the questions. Like Dante in the Fifth canto, I am overwhelmed. I fall.

Just as a dead body falls.

That phenomenon—contraction of the jaw muscles—was just the first in a long series in the years to come. Some were more painful, others less so. I always thought of them as being associated with moments of severe emotional stress, even though sometimes they just show up without any apparent reason. Nothing wrong with that—just one of the many compromises I have to live with. They are part of me and I've learned to accept them. They come and go without warning, and last just a few minutes. Sometimes I don't even pay attention to them. Sometimes they come at inopportune times, but somehow I manage to cope with them.

If the contraction happens during a conversation, I try to disguise it by distracting the other person, shifting her attention in other directions.

In fact, when I think about it, the most embarrassing situations I had to face were always at school. Whenever a contraction of the jaw muscles came right in the middle of an oral test, it was difficult to divert the teacher's attention. On those occasions, I was forced to counteract the muscular spasms with my hand, as I had done that fatal first time in class in high school, before I passed out. Sure, the teachers understood that something funny was happening to me. But who cared?

It was all part of a rather peculiar set.

A special person.

A real *rarity.*

The Professor's Hands

June 28th, 1985

Dear Diary,

Today is a very important day, and in a moment I'll tell you why. First of all, let me say that I just passed my school exams with an average A! Wonderful feeling, because I was not expecting it! And I was the only one in my class to get all As—can you believe that?

Well, school has been over for a bit, but there were not as many good-byes as I'd hoped. The girls from the other class disappeared almost immediately, whereas the rest of them, well, I barely had time to say hi. Alberto was very friendly and Ferdinando even shook my hand. I don't believe I'll ever forget him. I've dreamed about him every night since school finished. Ten nights in a row—I think I set a record!

But now we come to the most important fact of the day ... and of my whole life! Let's start all over again. On June 21st, last Friday, I went to Florence to be examined by a certain professor who is also a plastic surgeon, a scalpel wizard. I didn't really want to go, because I was tired of hanging around clinics, and I had made up my mind that I would stay as I am. But I went there and found myself immediately at ease because the receptionist was so kind. Then I entered the study for the examination and something happened that changed my whole life: the professor (a wonderful and very, very nice person!) told me that something can be done about my case, a form of plastic surgery that would improve my looks. This could be done either in September or even next week.

The professor told me that this way we could improve lip closure and said that I will even be able to kiss my boyfriend! It was all so sudden and so beautiful at the same time that it didn't seem real to me and I burst out crying. There and then I decided to have the operation in September, but once I was back home, thinking about it calmly, I decided to have it as soon as possible, in a week's time—that is, today.

This has been the most intense week of my life, no doubt about that, and today I'm a little scared because I'm not sure of the final outcome. Even though everyone is very encouraging, I'm a bit pessimistic as usual. Well, you can understand how important this day is. To think that tonight I'll be almost another person! Ok, well, hopefully.

Now I must leave you because it's 11:19 and I have to be there at 1pm sharp. Think of me and pray for me (so to speak). But I really really hope that those who love me will wish me all the luck in the world. I need it. Bye, I'll let you know.

Cristina

I even signed that diary entry, something I had never done before. Who knows, perhaps I just wanted to be certain it had really been me who had written those words and that I would not regret them in the future. Or perhaps it was a way to sign off on a part of my life that was about to end that morning, as by evening the doors would open to a new Cristina, one with another look, another life, perhaps even another signature.

I really believed it intensely. Despite my usually pessimistic nature, I truly had high hopes.

The professor had been recommended to us by friends-of-friends-of-friends-who-had-heard-say: a classic case of word of mouth, something you cling to like a castaway in times of need. Not that there was any urgent need for the surgery. As I wrote to my imaginary friend, after so much searching, looking, asking, I had decided to *stay as I am*. But whenever the hopes of my parents and my sisters were raised, I had to go with the flow. I couldn't just drop it. After all, it was not that hard for me to go a hundred more miles given all those I had travelled in the past.

In the mid–eighties, plastic surgery was still a largely unexplored world—at least for me—for us—it was. We had heard that it could "fix" a large and varied number of issues. We might as well try it. After all, until then, we had received an endless series of "noes," in every possible variation.

There is nothing we can do.

This issue can't be solved.

There is no solution.

No transplant.

No surgery.

Plastic surgery was an option we had not really considered before, and perhaps it would really be the turning point for my condition: maybe it would not solve the underlying issues, but at least it might improve my outward appearance, which in the past had attracted so much curiosity.

Today, I would not have remembered the *"kind receptionist,"* if I hadn't written those few words about her in my diary. The kind receptionist had the task of putting me in the right mood for the interview with the *"scalpel wizard,"* just like when you enter a room and the first thing you notice is a nice scent which predisposes you to positive feelings, erasing for a moment all other sensations. The kind receptionist had perfectly played the part of that "nice scent"—and yet, in spite of that, she was not destined to remain etched in my memory.

But the professor was.

I remember him so well. An imposing, gigantic, robust figure with a wide, toothy smile. And I remember his hands—enormous hands that, after a quick burst of shaking the hands of others for the required formal greetings, headed immediately towards my face, as if they were impatient to learn all its secrets. In the utter silence of the room, those hands investigated, analyzed, and studied every single inch of my visage. They pulled the skin, released it, and stretched it again, simulating the effects and the final results of the operation he was to perform.

"Yes, yes, yes. Let's see ... we will open here, shorten this part, take away this excess stuff here ... then you'll be able to close your mouth. You'll see, my dear, after the surgery you'll become a very pretty girl. Do you have a boyfriend? You'll find one, you'll find one, and how many kisses will you give him!"

My heart skipped a beat, my throat choked up, sounds refused to come out: of all the words the professor could have uttered in that solemn moment, he had chosen the most effective ones. He had touched one of the most delicate keys of my fragile emotional balance.

How could he have guessed my innermost thoughts? A thousand times I had wondered how I could ever kiss a boy if I was unable to close my lips, in what is the most natural act in the world for everybody else. Everybody else, yes, but not me. Me, I could only close my lips with a great, great effort, and usually with poor results.

I never dwelled too much on such thoughts, because I did not have definite answers. I could not even conceive of them—I was too scared to invent any solutions for that problem. So the most obvious escape was to relegate such thoughts, so hard to face, into a small corner of my brain, at the very bottom, in a dark and remote area difficult to reach. In the "taboo" section. Nobody would ever rummage in there unless I allowed them to.

And now, here comes this professor, this incredible solver of all the problems of the world, pulling the subject out of the hat with such enviable nonchalance, as if it were the most obvious, and the most evident, issue. The central problem that had troubled me so much, and that I had guarded jealously inside me, was an open secret to this man. And not just that: he even claimed to be able to help me solve it. He would eradicate the taboo with his own hands. Big, expert hands, the hands of *a wonderful and very, very nice person!*

A river of tears.

I remember them well too. Hot, salty, copious. I let them flow for a while. I was ashamed to let people see me like that, completely exposed, but I just could not help myself. Oh, no, I just couldn't. It was the outcome of all those long years of believing that no one could ever help me. No one.

But now the solution was right before me—imposing, wonderful and so very, very kind. The professor and his hands would finally save me from the emotional turmoil of my years, enormously magnified by my physical condition. I was more than sure about that. Someone who could guess people's most intimate secrets and most hidden taboos in such a natural way, well, he could not help but change your life once and for all. Could he not?

The professor and his hands did not change my life.

They did not even come close.

Just a week after our first meeting we had already set a date for the surgery. The decision had been taken following a few days of frantic debate mingled with overwhelming emotions. I have always been the kind of person who deals with issues headfirst, in a most direct manner, so as to get to the solution in the shortest possible time, and the prospect of months of uncertainty scared me a lot more than facing surgery very quickly. To wait until September was out of the question. If there had to be a revolution, then let it be soon.

Pronto!

The surgery was performed under local anesthetic in the professor's study and was not particularly difficult or painful. After a few hours' rest we were allowed to return home with the promise of meeting again at the next post-op check up. Luckily school was over and I had time to recover.

It took just a few days for me to realize that the general situation had barely changed, if at all. The lower lip had been shortened, but this did not bring any functional advantage. The difficulty of closing the lips was still there, and I surrendered to the idea that it would always be so.

No, the professor and his hands had not changed my life. They had just created two deep scars that would be with me forever. The first scar started from under my nose and crossed diagonally over my right cheek for a couple of inches; the second one was vertical, under the lower lip, shortening it by a few millimeters. The latter was particularly annoying because it did not heal in the time expected. As it was in a very delicate spot, I had to be careful not to overstretch the skin during meals; otherwise I would rip the stitches.

I was fed with liquids for at least a month after the surgery, but that did not matter to me. I could take it. Instead, what really worried me was that I had to live with new scars, this time physical and tangible, besides the interior ones, which were still there—invisible to all, but present nonetheless.

And yet there had been a change, an evolution.

People still looked at me (that would never change, no breakthrough from that point of view, definitely not), but unlike before they immediately took their eyes off me. The people I met finally seemed to *understand*. One of them even felt brave enough to formulate a question that at least had the merit of sounding new to my ears: "Did you have an accident?" Well, that was a good result in the end. Finally people were able to give themselves an explanation for my weird looks. The fresh scars on my face had assumed a peculiar function: they were reassuring, liberating, and explanatory.

I must certainly have suffered a serious accident, and what could be seen on my face was its sad aftermath.

People are scared of what they do not know and cannot explain with simple reasoning. People always want quick, easy and comforting answers. People want to have certainties. And so, from that day on, the scars on my face were my protection against prolonged, dumb, questioning stares. I would not be persecuted any more—or at least, not by everyone.

Of course the finger-pointing children were not discouraged by such good news: their endless morbid curiosity would not give up so easily. The finger-pointing children still existed and would exist forever and ever, until Judgment Day. But at least the grown-ups, who sometimes could be a thousand times more obtuse than any child, would now take their eyes off just one instant before their gaze became insistent.

But not all of them, not always.

I was already used to that. I was resigned. You cannot live with a cosmetic problem of any kind if you are unable to create a harmony within yourself. And from a certain point onward, curious stares no longer had any effect on me. Today I am sometimes even amused by them. When you grow up to learn that nobody, nobody in the whole world, has the right to make you feel like a rare species, obsessive stares must be accepted with just as much insistence, just as much obstinacy. And if this is not enough to deter such looks, you can even push yourself further, and ask with a candid tone, serene, as natural as possible, "Is there something wrong?" Usually this is the key question that makes everyone blush and puts people back in their place, implying that they have gone too far. Just a little bit.

To think back, these days, on how much I was hurt by those insistent stares only causes me a deep sense of loss. Every moment spent suffering for such nonsense was a wasted moment, lost forever.

It is a shame that I discovered this so late. But, of course, better late than never.

Spin the Bottle

All things considered, the last years in high school were flowing smoothly. I continued to experience those stupid and annoying contractions of the jaw muscles during oral tests, every now and then. I continued to accompany Laura, the indomitable leader, in improbable, unbearable, stressful, hilarious disco nights. I continued to get good grades and to avoid further temptations—read chatting with my desk-mate—I had moved two desks away from the root cause of my lively loquacity.

My powerful crush on Ferdinando was finally in a descending arc. I had long since realized that such a fixation would only bring painful disappointments; and in an attempt to save myself I tried to suppress my feelings as best I could, wishing above all to camouflage them from the eyes of my classmates. With little, decidedly little, results.

It was obvious to everyone how much I was actually attracted to him.

Deciding to physically stay away from Ferdinando during lessons had been a difficult yet necessary step. I was sure I would benefit a lot from it. It was never like that, of course, but at least I tried. None of my classmates, however, openly teased us. Everyone knew, but they left us alone in some sort of unspoken agreement, like, "You do not tease me, and I won't hate you for the rest of my life." Or something like that.

At least there had been an evolution, compared to that school trip, several years earlier, when our peers made fun of my feelings towards the boy I liked so much. At least my high school classmates had proven respectful towards other people's emotions, dignity and sensibility. Up to a point.

Until that night.

We had been invited to a birthday party, I don't even remember whose it was, since I considered them all equally depressing and boring. I always hated all forms of social gathering, as far back as I can remember, and teenage parties were a microcosm where I was not at all at ease. They constituted a smaller reproduction of what happened in

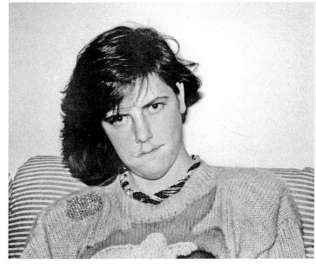

A pic taken at home on the day of my 17th birthday, 5 December 1987. The necklace I am wearing in the photograph was a birthday gift from my sisters.

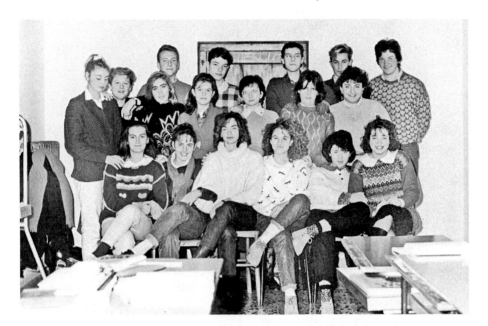

A pic of my high school class in Cortona, in the year 1988. Laura is the third from the right, in the front row, while Ferdinando is the fourth from the left at the top row, wearing a plaid sweater.

the endless nights spent at the disco: confusion, alienation, anxiety, boredom, and awareness of one's own uniqueness.

At class parties, the only difference was that we all knew each other, so—at least in theory—there would not be any reason for uneasiness. And yet, there was always some stranger there who ruined the evening and made me slip back into shyness and reservedness. Always.

That night, somebody had the splendid idea of playing spin the bottle, an extremely amusing party game that had facilitated all sorts of imaginative outpourings among young, naive and hormone-crazed teenagers for generations and generations. The teens sat in a circle around an empty bottle, somebody chose a forfeit, preferably a kiss on the cheek or where-you-like (just to be sure) and then spin the above-mentioned, treacherous bottle. And when it finally stopped, its neck inexorably pointed to the victim of the terrible forfeit.

It was hilarious, no doubt about it.

Unless you were afraid of being physically incapable of giving that fateful kiss.

Unless you thought that the victim in question did not really want to receive that fateful kiss from you.

The real forfeit, to me, was to have all those fears pile up in my head, all at once, all together. The real forfeit, to me, was to spin that damn bottle without knowing who would have to "suffer" my kiss. In ordinary life I used to stay away from embarrassing situations, so as to prevent them before they happened. That time, though, I could not escape my fate, since I was too ashamed to retreat from such a silly little game. I would only make things worse and attract even more attention to me—something I wanted to avoid at all costs.

Therefore, that night I could not save myself from the impending catastrophe. In any way.

The bottle spun, round and round, and finally pointed at me.

Someone gave me a kiss on the cheek, probably a female classmate, surely nobody compromising, otherwise I would remember. At that point it was my turn to put the infernal device in motion. I declared that my forfeit, surprise surprise, would be a kiss where-I-wanted (just to be sure). Nobody had anything to object to. Up to that point, nobody had complained about the monotonous choice of forfeits and nobody did in my case as well. The forfeit of the kiss-where-you-want (just to be sure) was all the rage that night, just like in a thousand other parties held by imaginative, original, tireless teenagers.

So, after my duty statement, I tried to give the bottle a good strong spin, while at the same time praying in silence that it would not end in the way I feared.

The circle comprised a dozen people: the chances of catastrophe happening were not so high, after all. And of course it happened—right on time. Like a slow-motion scene from some B-movie, I watched the bottle spin round and round and then wearily finish just where I didn't want it to—Ferdinando.

For a split second I estimated my chances of playing a magic trick: if I just concentrated as hard as I could perhaps I would have been able to disappear from sight and nobody would say anything, nor would they comment upon the disastrous result of that announced death sentence. And everyone would forever remember the miracle of my disappearance.

But the great Houdini did not come to my rescue, neither that night nor ever, and it took me a few embarrassing seconds to realize that inevitable, awkward truth.

Then someone spoke.

"Come on, give him a kiss! Everyone knows you were waiting just for that, weren't you?" Or something similar, equally horrendous.

I don't remember very clearly: at one point I think I just disconnected my brain—completely isolated from visions, sounds, smells. I believe that as in the best tradition the following phenomena ensued in this order: a hot flush in the face, accompanied by a diffuse redness of increasing intensity in the cheeks, tingling in the head, loss of feeling in the extremities of the body. To put it shortly, I was about to pass out.

Luckily, I had the promptness of spirit to get up and run away as fast as I could to another room, before becoming completely ridiculous, leaving behind a trail of vague bewilderment. I will never know what salacious comments followed on the part of my dear classmates. Actually, it is not something that has ever caused me sleepless nights, honestly. I bore a grudge for a few days towards the one who had casually thrown my dignity to the lions—that is, the entire class. After all, she had just voiced a simple, yet embarrassing truth.

Nowadays, I would think of a million different ways to react to such a situation. At eighteen, of course, none of them occurred to me. Better the classic retreat (just to be sure).

After that embarrassing night I was very cautious to keep a safe distance from Ferdinando—and from anyone who dared rehash what had happened. Fortunately, in a high school class there were new "epic" events more or less daily, and so the "spin the bottle" story was soon relegated to the basement of all my classmates' memories, next to hundreds of equally succulent anecdotes that occurred during our five years of cohabitation.

There were no particular consequences from that event, not even veiled hints: my nonrelationship with Ferdinando remained as such until the end of school, with no major events worthy of note.

And, to quote Forrest Gump, that's all I have to say about that.

The Monster in Room 204

Malice is something I could never stand, and I am certainly not the intolerant type. When you are lacking a certain aesthetic appeal, you tend to compensate for its loss with the right amount of inner charisma, if we can call it that. You strive to seem more nice and sympathetic than you actually are, you try to be more accommodating with the next man, and most of all you get to be more tolerant.

The key word here is "compromise." In life, I have always been ready to come to all sorts of compromises, from the most insignificant to the heaviest. Anything not to annoy others, anything to be accepted by them, as best as I could, always. What is more, hardly ever anyone tries to make a nice gesture for somebody who is not pleasant-looking. I know it is sad to say, but it's a fact. It never happened that somebody helped me lift up my suitcase onto a train compartment rack, for instance. Never. Either I have been very unfortunate in my traveling experiences, or it is a cruel reality. I would incline for the second hypothesis.

So, no niceties in sight for ugly girls. I can accept this. I said it before: I am tolerant.

I am also ready to accept another major scourge of our century: indifference. There are people who simply act and behave as if you just were not there—in that moment, in that room, in that universe. And that's fine for me. I can understand it. I can tolerate it.

But malice, no way. Pure wickedness is a condition I cannot and will not accept in any form. It is neither explainable nor justifiable. Malice is just execrable, nothing more than that. It is shocking, terrible, and obscene.

It is a very serious disease that grips the mind—thank goodness—of only a few. Still, those few can cause countless damage. I happened to come across malice three times during my life. A rather low score perhaps, but one that marked me forever. All three episodes date back to my high school years; when I was old enough to understand that they could not be misinterpreted but not strong enough to be able to assimilate them, embrace them, accept them. They were all embarrassing, painful and cruel moments, in that order.

This is their story.

One

My high school had organized a special one-day trip to the mountains. Mount Abetone, a couple of hours from home, is the one of the most important ski resorts in the Apennines. I was attending the third year and was one of the few in my class who could ski. I never thought that there were things that not everyone was able to do, and it was a nice surprise to discover that I had skills not available to many of my peers. I mentally thanked my sisters, who used to take me with them, ever since I was a little girl, on their holidays in the snow with their "big" friends and allow me to learn a sport that was not at all common in our region.

That day I felt good, strong, and capable.

Nothing in the world could bring me down from that tiny little pedestal that I had created for myself, and on which I had climbed up for once in my life, leaving the others below me—just a little bit, but more than enough.

I strapped on my skis and headed for one of the ski lifts. Every now and then I met some people I knew, even if only by sight, and ventured so far as to greet them first. An absolute novelty for me, as I was usually afraid of not being reciprocated, and therefore always avoided that kind of risk. That day, everyone responded to my greetings.

I was skiing with pleasure, and in a particularly difficult descent I experienced one of those moments that I called "mystical," where I found myself thinking that living was really a beautiful thing. It occurred to me only rarely to have such absolutely positive thoughts about life. That day, at that moment, I thought I finally understood what happiness meant.

Then it happened.

I was passing near two teenage boys who were sitting down to fix their boots. Both, like me, were obviously skilled in skiing. One of them I knew only by sight: he was attending the final year at high school and was a classmate of a very good friend of mine since childhood. The other boy near him was my dear childhood friend. He lived in the same village where I had spent the first few carefree years of my life, just a few yards from my parents' house. He was also the best friend of my legendary cousin, the one who had protected me from all the bad kids. Therefore he was someone I really loved and with whom I had played so many times in the past.

I raised my hand to greet him while slipping by in the snow beside them. He smiled at me and nodded. Then the other guy made a comment.

"I didn't know mongoloids could ski."

He said those words in a low voice, thinking I could not hear him. But the message arrived loud and clear, and it hit the mark. I had a painful pang in my heart. But it was nothing compared to the one that was about to come, after my childhood friend replied, also thinking I wouldn't hear.

"Me neither."

I didn't turn back, didn't slow down, and didn't stop. I simply carried on. I felt numb and it took me a few seconds to regain control of my breathing, heartbeat and leg muscles. I felt betrayed in an irreparable way. If I could not even count on a friendship rooted in mutual knowledge and trust, how could I ever expect to find a true friend? If even those people I believed were on my side abandoned me at the first hurdle, what hope could I have in the future?

I would always be a freak to laugh at, without any chance that someone would take my side. I would be alone to fight my fight. Without friends or external aid. There were no real values—only so much dryness.

And sadness.

Two

What a wonderful birthday party Laura had organized! Her parties were always epic, no doubt about that. The funniest, the headiest and the most exciting. Her birthday was the event that everyone looked forward to: since she was born in June, it also marked the end of another heavy school year. To celebrate her and with her gave us all a sense of mutual joy, as if her party had become our own. From that day on, only freedom and fun were awaiting us.

As far as I was concerned, Laura's parties were the only ones where I found myself completely at ease. Nothing like those organized by the other classmates, which I always faced with a certain pent-up anxiety. She made me feel as though her home were mine, since we had known each other for a lifetime. Being born in the same village, we obviously had the same acquaintances—not only schoolmates, old and new alike, but also all our peers who had grown up with us but were attending different schools.

That day, for her eighteenth birthday, Laura had arranged a special party and invited a flood of people, including a boy, older than us, who had been at the center of a small drama inside our class. Two of my classmates, best friends since elementary school, had found themselves attracted to the same boy, who had graciously agreed to start a relationship with both, at the same time, without either of them being aware of the fact.

This classic love triangle, as tradition dictated, had ended in the worst possible way: hysterical arguments, embarrassing scenes of jealousy in front of the whole class, and a friendship truncated in a permanent and definitive way, despite all those years the two girls had spent together like twin sisters.

The episode disturbed the whole class, since we all knew the two protagonists and found it hard to believe that such a strong friendship could be wiped out in a heartbeat for a reason so futile. And yet one of the most important unwritten laws had been violated, one that every eighteen-year-old girl knows very well: thou shalt not covet thy neighbor's boyfriend—especially mine.

All this for him. For this boy who now, at Laura's party, I finally had the chance to meet. At last.

It was the first time I saw the "big guy." He was the idol our imaginations had turned into mythical proportions, the one who had succeeded in destroying such an indissoluble friendship, and now he was standing in front of me. He was talking to one of my classmates and they seemed to be having a jolly good time. I immediately felt a bit of discomfort. First of all, he was not the Adonis I had imagined. He looked ugly. I just couldn't understand what not just one, but two of my prettiest classmates had found so attractive in him.

Oh, well, you know, *each to his own*. After all, who was I to judge—

But those eyes—black, hostile, dangerous. Cold and at the same time malignant. I never thought I would be able to recognize evil at first sight— it had never happened to me before. Still, now I had it right in front of me: clear, patent, frightening.

It was like my inner defenses had woken up and all the alarms had been activated. I tried to stay away from him as much as possible. Somewhere inside me, I was aware of what could happen if he focused on my person and my condition. For a while I succeeded. Then, inevitably, those eyes that I had tried to avoid throughout the day noticed my existence. And just as I'd predicted, the great guy, the womanizer, had no better notion than to externalize his deepest and innermost thoughts, sharing them with the whole community of my friends and classmates. Pointing his finger at me, a gesture that seemed to emerge straight from the depths of my past, he formulated the question.

"Who the hell is *this*? Does anyone know her? Did she crawl straight out of Loch Ness?"

A moment of silence and general embarrassment ensued.

It is true that my instinct had warned me not to expect good things from that guy, but not anything so damn bad.

I did not think I deserved so much attention. I did not think there were still pointing-finger kids aged 20. And I did not think such a pure form of treachery could exist. That day, after making all those discoveries, I felt hurt, for the umpteenth time, without anyone to blame. What bad people don't realize is that it is not fun to be different, and diversity is never a desired choice. It is a condition that we find ourselves in without having asked for it. We try to hide it as best as we can so as not to annoy the odd "big guy," but sometimes we just can't.

That's why I prefer indifference to wickedness. Being invisible to other people's eyes causes sadness, but at least it does not expose one to ridicule and embarrassment.

Since that day, over the years I have had the chance to meet this most desired womanizer a number of times. I continue to avoid him, even though today I would have some answers to his questions.

Anyway, he still looks ugly to me—hideous, I'd say. But, you know, *each to his own*—

And his eyes are always the same. Terrible, chilling and inhuman.

And that's a fact.

Disputandum non est.

Three

The summer holidays following our high school's final exams were very intense, lived moment by moment and enjoyed all the way, a well-deserved period of rest after months of study and stress leading to the most difficult exams in every student's life. That year, as usual, Rimini was our family's destination, together with Laura and her family, to forget the labors of school and restore our energy.

We immediately met a group of friends at our hotel, who "adopted" us with great enthusiasm. The group was quite varied, with many boys and girls from all parts of Italy. While Laura made victims among the boys, I became good friends with a girl from Bolzano, same age as us, who worked as a nurse. We used to hang out together, and for the entire period of our holiday I never had the feeling that something was not going the right way. Of course most of the boys ignored me completely, but that was fine with me as I was used to it. Good ol' indifference.

Upon returning home I stayed in touch with the nurse for several months, through the mail: we told each other small episodes of our daily life.

Then, one day, I received a letter with no return address. According to the postmark it came from Pavia, in Northern Italy. I seemed to recall that three boys from our holiday group came from that town, but I was not too sure, since I never talked to any of them. We just cheerfully ignored each other, or so it seemed to me.

A little curious and a bit puzzled, I opened the letter.

It was typewritten, and went like this:

Rimini: The day after.
It was a seemingly quiet day, the one the three boys were about to live.
The day before the extraordinary event the three friends had heard a

floating of indefinite masses in a room of their hotel, causing strange currents that could lift a crocodile off the ground.

The fateful room was on the second floor and our heroes walked towards the origin of such a powerful stench. Armed with a lot of courage, they approached Room 204.

The stench that came out of it was unimaginable, and from it also stemmed a source of fluorescent and flashing light that kept increasing in intensity as the brave boys approached. When they reached the "X" spot they looked at each other and opened the door.

The sight was horrible: a greenish monster, with no eyes but with a huge mouth that uttered ghastly and incomprehensible noises stood in the middle of the room. Then it started moving towards them...

End of first part

Fantomax fan club

There was no doubt who played the part of the greenish monster. And just in case I had any, they would be dispelled by the fact that the room I had occupied at the hotel in Rimini was number 204. After reading that letter, I was annihilated. I could not figure out where so much hatred, so much ill will and so much contempt came from.

Those three boys, well, I barely noticed them during the holidays, and realizing that they had spent a lot of time and effort to locate my address, find out my surname and concoct that nasty little story, made me feel dizzy. They had to gather, search, and devise, put into practice. How much wickedness was needed to come up with such a plan, organized in every detail? It seemed unbelievable that they would waste their time in such a stupid way. Unbelievable and cruel. Brutal. Evil. Senseless.

From that day on I stopped looking for answers to some questions.

Wickedness is a fact. It does not have to be justified. It exists and hurts, but after sparking a moment of astonishment in you it leaves you the time to assimilate it and fight back—always.

The second part of that elaborate horror story never arrived. Perhaps my three friends from Pavia had found a new hobby to pass their days. Or a new victim to harass.

Because one thing is for sure: wickedness is a beast with certain common characters. A smelly, creepy, fluorescent greenish being with no eyes. But with a huge mouth that would always be hungry.

These episodes meant a lot to me. They showed me the dark side of people, but they also helped me understand. They led me to reflect on the contrary. Usually one tends to notice always and only the negative episodes, the people who look at you and make comments in a low voice, those who ignore you or despise you at first sight.

But for each of them there are hundreds, thousands of people who accept you, open up to you and your diversity.

Human wickedness is absurd and inexplicable, but purity of mind is equally incredible. And fortunately it is much more frequent and easier to find.

Sometimes I think that my peculiarity, my uniqueness, is so evident that even I would find it difficult to ignore it altogether were I to be "on the other side." Still, it often occurs that people do not pay attention to it at all. And not because they are making an effort to hide their surprise, but just because they are not interested in difference. What matters to them is to dig deeper, beyond the wall of aesthetics, and go directly to the soul and the heart of a person.

Isn't that a *rarity* just as amazing? It is, of course it is.

Life confronts us with all kinds of people, and over the years I have learned to appreciate this variety, this daily challenge in meeting someone. We have to allow ourselves to accept any human type, since every human being is entitled to a chance.

And we have to give it to them. Whatever the cost.

Eighteen

Turning eighteen definitely changed a number of things in my life. First of all, it made me a bit more responsible and forced me to do by myself certain tasks that until then had been taken care of by my parents.

I met my first small difficulty after coming of age at the city hall's registry office the day I went there to have my first ID card. I had begged my mom to come with me, but—being well aware that it was the right time to let me cope with the twisted labyrinth of bureaucracy—she flatly refused. She added that I knew how to express myself very well for such a simple request, and I would be perfectly able to take care of myself.

I had not insisted she go, since I didn't want to disappoint her. Still, my usual shyness prevented me from facing such news all by myself, in one single day, all of a sudden. Anyway, I was not going to give up at the first difficulty.

First, I plucked up the courage and went to a photographer, to have my pictures taken. The pictures, indeed. Another frightening obstacle to deal with. It had already happened before, and I had to succumb to the need of having my awkward image immortalized in an ID photo. Each time it had been a nightmare: as soon as I got in position, invariably the photographer would urge me to make a nice smile.

Ah, Ah. Sure. Good joke.

You know, Mr. Photographer, I'd like to make not just one smile but two, ten, a thousand. But I'm afraid they would not look too good.

Of course I couldn't even look the photographer in the eyes due to my embarrassment, let alone answer him that way. I just did my best, with a grimace that I tried to make as close as possible to something resembling a smile, with a huge effort from my nonexistent muscles and nonfunctioning nerves—and totally useless.

After a few seconds, the photographer surrendered to the fact that my face would not generate anything and used his infernal device, which, after the customary "click," regurgitated the product of so much suffering. A picture of horror or—when things went very, very well—merely antipathy. But that was me, and that was what I had to make do with, with all due respect to my instinctive feelings of revulsion.

That day I did not fare any better: the same scene repeated itself just like the other times—embarrassing, unpleasant, depressing. However, I picked up the four pictures, all identical and ugly, and made my way to the registry office of my small town.

There were lots of people in line before me, and the wait seemed to go on endlessly. During all that time, I mentally repeated the phrase with which I would introduce myself as soon as my turn arrived. I repeated it over and over, obsessively. Always the same, again and again, as if for fear of forgetting a part of it.

"Hello, I'm here to make my ID card."

Difficult. Insidious. But carefully chosen, so that there would be as few labials as possible. Oh, well, there were still a few, but within the general context I hoped they would be comprehensible. Finally my turn came.

"Hello. ID card."

No labials! I won! I had out-smarted *them*.

The clerk on duty glanced at me for a moment and made his move. He was certainly the boss of *them* all. The more cunning and astute. And he was surely trying to set me up with that enigmatic, devious request.

"Your name and surname, please."

Ok, even though I feel this is a trap I'm going to tell you. But mind you that I am well aware that you are trying to confuse me—all of *you*.

"Cristina Faragli."

He looked up, staring at me, puzzled.

"Sorry—what?"

Uhm, ok, be calm and try again. Perhaps I didn't make myself clear. Perhaps there was too much noise.

Perhaps it's all a plot, but I'll try again all the same.

"Cristina Faragli."

This time he looked a bit more impatient.

"I don't understand."

Okay, now I'm saying it less vehemently. Perhaps that's what distracted him—vehemence.

"Cristina Faragli."

He made a funny grimace, to make it clear to me that he didn't get it, not even this time.

"*Saragli?*"

Uh, there it was. All clear, at last. The damned *F*. And now, what am I supposed to do? I could stand here all day and he would not understand—*none* of them would. Now or ever. Then, the illumination came. So obvious and yet so late.

"Faragli. F like Florence."

His face lit up, the light at the end of the tunnel.

"Oh, there we are! How come it took so long?"

Mortified and a little downcast, I answered his questions without any major hitches. At the end of that morning I was holding in my hands a brand new ID card and had a bit of confusion in my mind; but in my heart I knew for sure that the world, the so-called civil society, would not be kind to me in the future. There were still many such walls of obtuseness for me to climb. Walls built by all of *them*, with method and expertise.

But there was another thing I was sure of: the phrase "F like Florence" would become my ally for many, many occasions to come.

And I wasn't wrong. Not at all.

There was a specific reason in desiring to reach the legal age as soon as possible. I wanted a driving license. I had been longing for it for so many years, and I had been practicing my driving, from the time I was little more than a child. There was a large yard in front of my house that was ideal for my first forays as a reckless car driver. I started driving a car at 12, even before I was given a scooter. My parents did not find anything wrong in my having some fun "playing" with mom's yellow Fiat 500. On Sundays, with the yard clear of other vehicles all just for me, I practiced with my sisters, who in turn served as instructors in the next seat.

Driving has always given me a sense of freedom and profound joy, especially on those occasions when I was allowed to explore the nearby country roads when there was no traffic, which in practice meant mostly weekends. I found it so natural to learn how to drive a car that I often asked myself why it was legally permitted only to citizens aged 18 or older.

The wait looked like an eternity, but I finally got there. I attended the lessons of theory and practice at the local driving school and received the instructor's compliments. During driving lessons, I had to curb my instincts as an experienced pilot, as they would not be appreciated. I had to be careful and cautious, never exceeding thirty miles an hour, for one thing. It was torture, but I was ready to undergo any kind of self-restriction in order to have my final exams as soon as possible.

So, after just eight driving lessons, the minimum allowed by law, I was ready for the final exams. The theory tests had been a success, as I knew all the quizzes by heart, having practiced them so many times at home, by myself, exercising for the final test. However, I needed just one more thing to be able to access the driving test itself: a certificate from the medical health department.

It was a very simple eye examination, to ensure that my eyesight was adequate to the required standards. Fortunately I never had problems in that area: 20/20 in each eye, although the doctors were never able to explain such an anomaly compared to those typical of the Moebius Syndrome. Usually, in fact, the syndrome causes many problems to the eyesight, in various ways. Those affected by it are usually unable to move their eyes laterally, and other typical characters include strabismus and extreme eye sensitivity (a pathology which marginally affected me). But at least I had been spared that particular corollary.

I went to the examination in a rather agitated mood and could not explain why. My sight was perfect, there was no reason to worry. Still, I felt a sense of inner discomfort: perhaps my subconscious, always prepared for the worst, was sending warning signs.

Deep down, even though I did not want to admit it to myself, I was afraid that my congenital syndrome would make the difference. I tried to convince myself that it was a silly thought, because in this case there was absolutely no relationship between the malfunctioning of my facial muscles and the driving license I wanted so much to achieve. There was no other point on which to object: my legs, arms, heart and eyes were perfectly functional, and I would not need anything else to drive. Nevertheless, my eternally pessimistic nature was working frantically, warning me from every possible eventuality.

I was agitated. I was shaking. I was scared.

On the morning of the test, my mother accompanied me, but when my turn came I told her I wanted to go in alone. I wanted to show her that I had already developed a remarkable self-confidence, the one she wanted me to show after I turned eighteen.

I stayed in there less then two minutes.

I had hardly introduced myself before the health physician had already decided that I was the carrier of a serious case of dementia. After merely a first, superficial glance he had taken the drastic decision not to give me any chance. He blathered about I-don't-know-what-kind-of-technical impossibility: he made a brief mention of the difficulties of that specific case and away, next please, we're done here.

I could not utter a single word.

My mother, seeing me coming out of the office so early, immediately sensed what might have happened. It was not necessary to explain anything. She knew there would be need of her intervention. She was quite good at that. Very, very good. Especially when it came to fight for me against all the injustices of the world. It all happened in a few seconds. She put on her invisible armor—invisible to everyone but me, who distinctly perceived its blazing fire-red color—and stepped inside the office. Alone.

I sat there, awaiting events. Other people waiting for their turn were staring at me, perplexed. They felt there had been some kind of hitch but could not imagine what it might be. Floating in a sea of embarrassment, I just did not know what to do. Eyes fixed on the floor, I sat waiting for inhuman yells to come out of that room at any moment.

And yet, all was quiet. After ten minutes of silent battle, my mom came out, looking absolutely radiant. She took me by the hand, greeted all the people in the waiting room, wished them a good day, and dragged me away from that nightmare.

In her hand she held two papers. The first was the report card of my senior year at the high school. I was puzzled.

"Mom, what were you doing with *that*?"

She stopped, looked me straight in the eyes and uttered the words that would stay inside me forever and ever, branded in fire on my heart.

"The world is packed full with ignorant people. Ignorance can overcome anything. That doctor's superficiality comes from his ignorance. We must always be prepared to prevent ignorance from beating you. I knew I had to prove your intelligence with something tangible, like a document, and I brought it in with me, just in case.

Never allow anyone to think they're better than you!

You have to fight to defend your intelligence.

You have to fight to shout your qualities to the world.
You have to bite if you don't want to be bitten."
I would never forget those words.
She gave me a kiss and handed me the second paper—the certificate of fitness to drive.

Two

Learning to Fly

Veni Vidi Vinci

We left the last turn behind us and I finally saw it, right in front of me. I had heard so many things about it that I could say I already knew it well: the village where my sisters had done their studies in optics. Optics was a fascinating subject taught in very few institutes throughout the country, and the most prestigious of all was right there, in the very heart of Tuscany, the hometown of the great Renaissance genius, Leonardo. The town of Vinci. And there we were, after a two-hour drive. Tiziana asked me a question but I did not reply, lost as I was in my thoughts.

"So, Cri, are you ready for this new adventure?"

Was I? A weird yet positive feeling had caught me after that last turn. I felt a small pang. The main square reminded me of the one where I grew up many years earlier. And the institute—that massive yellow building, perfectly symmetrical, right in the main square—immediately aroused a magnetic attraction in me.

I liked it there, I definitely did. And I finally answered my sister's question.

"Yes, I think I'm ready."

After finishing high school I had the chance to choose my future: either to attend the college or to follow in the footsteps of my older sisters, who had studied at Vinci and opened an optical shop in town.

Every year Vinci accommodated students from all over Italy, to the joy of the villagers—and their pockets. Many of them had adapted their own homes and used to rent rooms to young people from every part of the peninsula. Not only that, the prestige of the IRSOO School of Optics and Optometry was such that it drew many foreign students as well, given that the final graduation would be effective also in their country of origin.

I had already savored a taste of the atmosphere that was breathed in Vinci, the times when I came there to visit my sisters during their stay in the town. I was only seven years old then, but I had already sensed that it was a special place, where strong bonds would grow between people who would always remain in each other's lives, as had happened with Rossella and Tiziana. My sisters were still in touch with their old IRSOO schoolmates, who regularly came to pay us visits from all over Italy. It was a fascinating thing, and it could happen to me as well, maybe. It was well worth trying.

A few days before leaving for Vinci, I started a new diary. I wanted to fix on paper the feelings and emotions I was about to experience so I would remember them forever. My stay at Vinci might turn up as a fleeting experience, a matter of just a few days before I would realize that it would not be the beginning of a new life. On the other hand, it might well develop into an adventure waiting to be discovered—and an opportunity to achieve my two most intimate desires.

The first was to find a best friend who could at least compete with the role Laura had played up to that point.

Second, and above all, was to meet a boy who would accept me for what I was, with all my physical shortcomings included in the package.

I started the diary in a moment of deep inner reflection, expressing the mood of those days, as if I wanted to summarize in a few lines the gloomy feelings that had been flooding my soul for some time and were tormenting me so, more and more frequently.

No "Dear diary" as the opening words here, no funny lines. I had grown up. I had become mature. No jokes, either. Only thoughts put on paper in a stream of consciousness filled with pessimism.

> I'm going through a particularly difficult time of my life.
> I think it is called "identity crisis," but whatever the name is, it certainly does not help me to have a serene life. More and more often lately I stop to think what the hell I came into this world for, and what purpose can my life have. It is very difficult for me to understand why I was born, since up to now my life has not given me much happiness ... quite the contrary, actually. I must say that the fact of not being "normal" really affects me a lot, and never allows me to be completely, one-hundred-percent happy.
> I am sure that the actual condition will not improve in the future, and above all I am worried that I will always be alone for the rest of my life, since I will never find someone who'll have the courage to spend his life next to "somebody" like me.
> Until now I have been brave and consoled myself with my family's love, which is immense, but often this is not enough for me any more. That's why I'm starting to envy Enzo.

I have noticed that since his accident I don't have the fear of dying that I once had. The idea of ending like him does not upset me perhaps because I would avoid living painful and miserable years, carrying an increasingly heavy burden.

Yes, sure, but how could I do that? Death should come naturally; I could never bring it on myself in a mechanical way. Never. So, how do I find the strength to carry on?

Somebody help me, please.... I need a reason to live.

I just hope that the new school will give me a bit of happiness, a break from all this anguish. I don't think I'm asking too much.

Enzo was a friend of mine who had passed away the year before after a terrible motorcycle accident. He was seventeen. We were the same age, had attended elementary and middle school together, and he had been Laura's very first boyfriend, at a time when "being together" meant going to school hand in hand. He was one of the many friend-brothers of those early happy childhood years when I had lived in a serene, carefree way. His death upset me deeply and made me think for the first time about the true meaning of life. From then on, whenever I felt bad I thought about him and how easy it would be to leave everything behind, with no regrets. Forever.

Identity crisis.

Maybe.

Or simply infinite weariness. Alienation. Then, however, it disappeared. At least for some time. Until the next crisis. In spite of the desired *one-hundred-percent* happiness.

In order to access the courses at Vinci's IRSOO, it was necessary to attend an admission test. On the day, I woke up charged and determined: my life would take a decisive turn following that test, and the thought excited me so much.

Tiziana and I drove the hundred miles that separated us from Vinci, talking about her school memories. Then we drove past that last turn. It was the first time that I had been away from home for a prolonged period. I was overwhelmed by doubts, but at the same time I was curious to see how I would cope with them.

We arrived early in the morning, and sat on the marble stairs outside the institute, waiting for our turn to go in. I saw many boys and girls my age coming over, all looking a bit disoriented. Some were with their parents, many others were alone. In the midst of them, I noticed one girl, in particular, who wore a pair of Ray-Ban sunglasses identical to mine. She was sitting all alone, waiting like all of us for the school door to open. Finally, after a few more minutes, we were allowed to enter and, waving to my sister, I walked towards my destiny.

There were a lot of us, about 120 boys and girls all facing the test, and I began to have doubts about all of us passing it. I sat in one of the first rows and started to take out of my bag the pens and pencils I would use during the test when I felt a finger tapping me on my shoulder. I turned back and found myself facing the beaming smile of the girl with the Ray-Ban sunglasses.

"Hi, I'm Donatella, and you?"

I could not believe that. Somebody was interested in me and even wanted to know who I was—an absolute novelty up until that moment.

"Hi, I'm Cristina."

And I believe we will become good friends, I had thought at the same time.

Best friends.

"I've seen you outside the school, Cristina. I really like your cardigan sweater, I have one which is very similar, you know?"

Same tastes, too. No doubt, I had found a friend.

Despite my preoccupations, I passed the test. The next step was to find accommodation. With my sister's help, I rented a room right next to the school, a comfortable cozy place that I would share with two other girls. They chose a double room next to mine. I took a single one. Integration, yes, but little by little, please. To share an apartment was one thing, but sleeping in the same room with a total stranger was a step too far for the moment.

My first impression of Vinci had been positive, thanks in large part to Donatella, her sunglasses, and her smile, and I looked forward to the promise of pleasant days spent together.

I came home very confident about my future. In fact, I could not wait to start that adventure.

One-Hundred-Percent

Since my first days in Vinci I realized that such an experience would be the turning point of my life. In class I sat next to Donatella: a great fellowship immediately grew between us, both in study and, especially, our free time. Donatella had a certain charisma, and it did not bother me at all. Our new friends seemed to accept me the same way they approached her, with extreme ease. I never felt out of place: we were all part of a nice group of friends who used to share every moment, in education and in entertainment. The fact of being somehow forced to live side by side in the same place made us very close to one another, and for the first time in my life I experienced what being part of a group—of a *whole*—meant.

We used to go out almost every night, and sometimes we would gather at one of our friends' places, or else we took the car and hit some pub in the nearby towns, or we simply met in the main square and talked about school, marks, teachers, and our new life.

There was one episode in particular, Nancy, which made me smile. It happened one of the first times we were in the main square, chatting, after school. I was with Donatella and some other friends, all of them new faces I would begin to know very well a little later. We were sitting on a bench, and a cute boy I had glimpsed during lessons sat next to me. I did not even know his name.

He said he was a bit cold, especially in the hands, and with a disarming naturalness he asked me if I did not mind warming them up with mine. An utterly normal request, but with a huge meaning for me. Never, never, never before had any boy spontaneously wanted to have physical contact with me—of any kind, ever.

And now this stranger, this wonderful specimen of the male gender, with his cute northern accent, declared his intention to establish contact. Physical contact. With me.

I do not know what his thoughts were when he noticed that I was staring at him. For a few seconds I kept looking at the guy, trying to figure out whether he was simply kidding or, even worse, trying to tease me, luring me into a trap of some kind. I was so slow to respond to his request, my mind lost in endless doubts, that I did not even notice that my hands were already caught between his. He was holding them tightly, as if they were a precious object which could instill a never-ending warmth.

I shifted my gaze in disbelief from his eyes to our intertwined hands. And then again to his eyes. He was smiling, and in that moment I thought I was living the happiest moment of my whole life. Of course it did not mean anything: a simple gesture of human kindness which I was not used to. But to me, it meant everything.

It was the beginning of a new and wonderful experience.

Friends who did not sense my particular condition as a problem would surround me. I felt accepted, a member of that new community, finally useful and important, just like any *normal* human being. I was thrilled. I was beginning to think that there would be some interesting developments in my future. I was convinced that staying in Vinci would be the only opportunity to turn myself into a happy person.

One-hundred-percent happy.

A few months later there was a new episode, unique and unexpected.

Well, I never thought that I would be sitting here at 2:54 in the morning, writing in my diary.

Yet it is so. I wanted to do it right away because everything is still fresh in my mind and I wish I could convey what I have in my heart onto the page.

I found a male friend! A TRUE friend.

We've been a couple of hours in his car, talking about personal issues and the most important thing for me is that at the end of the evening he thanked me for existing!

He said that I am very important to him and that if he ever has any problems he will immediately come over and confide only in me! This fact could be meaningless to anyone else, but to me it is so important.

To me, who never had a male friend.

To me, who had always been rejected by all.

To me, who now and then think it would be better to die.

From now on I have a friend. I wish it was forever.

Most important, very important, so important.

I had obsessively repeated this concept three times in a few lines. And it really was important to me. It was finally the time to start getting out of that cocoon in which I was born and grew up, made up of layers and layers of distrust towards the whole human race. I had found somebody who appreciated my qualities as a listener, and to me it was already an extraordinary event. Even the simple fact that the boy had given me the chance to express myself, my inner self, instead of stopping at aesthetic impressions, seemed miraculous. He listened to me, understood me, and felt the desire to confide in me, in turn.

Unbelievable.

Never before had I experienced so confidential and intimate an exchange of views with a boy, a representative of the opposite sex. The only experience that could be compared to it was the school trip to Rome. Maybe. *Very vaguely.* But that innocent one-to-one dialogue with Ferdinando had been nothing compared to this. And yet I had not fallen in love with my new friend.

I was growing up. And I had stored in my mind the information that it's not always necessary to fall for someone who's paying attention to you. There already had been the episode of the intertwined hands, and even then I hadn't built any strange illusion on the event. That evening— or rather, that night—I realized that a simple friendship could result in a feeling of immense inner warmth. Perhaps not as great as the one you would expect from a love story, but I would make do with it for the time being.

Or so I hoped.

To obtain a certificate of qualification to practice as an optician, it was enough to attend the lessons of only one of the three academic years in the program. Some of my classmates decided to stop at that point. Me, I was determined to spend the next two years at Vinci, to fully exploit the immense amount of information that I could still learn from the experience.

The choice of continuing that fabulous adventure was spontaneous. The idea of interrupting it prematurely did not even occur to me. I felt good in that small town, within that varied, heterogeneous community made up of friends from all over Italy and abroad. I never dreamed of feeling so at ease in a place that only a little while before had been completely alien to me. For nothing in the world would I give up the chance of spending two more years with my new friends. For nothing and no one in the whole world.

The Butterfly Effect

In June, at the end of the first school year, I felt so involved in my optical studies that I did not miss the opportunity to attend, after lessons had ended, a course in contactology that had been scheduled in the next few days. The course would last only a couple of weeks—fifteen days more to savor in Vinci before the summer holidays began. I could not miss it.

Donatella also decided to stay two weeks more to attend the course. It is likely we planned it together, as we did all the important decisions in that school year. The thought of having to stay apart for a whole long summer was devastating for both of us. For that reason, we tried to stretch out our school experience as much as possible, and the course in contactology was a perfect excuse, coming at just the right moment.

During the course, the relationship with our teachers intensified exponentially. The topic was the study of contact lenses: how they were made, what materials they were made of, the way they had to be applied on the patients' eyes.

This last part was the funniest: we divided into small groups of two, and each one practiced on the other applying contact lenses. Each day the couples would change, and this way we soon became buddies—we had to, or else there would be a chance of getting somebody else's unwanted finger in the eye.

Two unforgettable weeks, during which I got to know for the first time some of those classmates I had not previously hung out with. New friendships that brought new joy in my life.

The course in contactology united us in an indissoluble way: sticking fingers in each others' eyes created an inevitable bond, as well as a certain intimacy, so to speak. We often said it as a joke, but deep down we knew it was really like that: staying still, motionless, eyes wide open, waiting for a contact lens to be applied was a small act of faith, a way to be of service to our classmates and declare our own trust in them—hoping that the trust would be rewarded. That meant trying not to shed copious, warm tears immediately after the application—which nevertheless promptly happened every time—to everyone. But we cried happily, glad to help our companion, who was going to learn more or less quickly, depending on how patient we were under such torture.

Patient: a magic word.

Here's where the meaning came from. Now everything was clear.

I understood it that summer, during the course in contactology in Vinci.

The most *patient* patient of all my classmates was a Greek boy, Vassilis.

The Hellenic community was rather large in the town of Vinci and, understandably, it formed a group of its own. Visibly present, but mostly invisible to our eyes. Vassilis, or "Vas" as we called him, was extremely shy, spoke little or very little during the course, and above all, never complained. He was the perfect guinea pig.

Despite his introverted nature, we exchanged some bits of conversation every now and then, and I discovered that he had enrolled at the school of optics very late. Lessons had started in early October, when he was still learning the basics of the Italian language at the school for foreigners in Perugia.

Vassilis had left his small Greek village without knowing what awaited him. In Perugia he found a girlfriend, Ioanna, a Greek girl who had also recently arrived in Italy, to study pharmacy. Then someone told him about the IRSOO in Vinci. He left Perugia and enrolled at the school over a month and a half after lessons had started. The first impression had been tough: he hadn't found a single vacant room in town, and for him it was back and forth from the town of Empoli, every day, on the bus, at impossible hours.

It seemed to me that he had enormous courage, and I admired him so much, unconditionally. I had put myself in his shoes and realized I would never have the same tenaciousness, perseverance and stubbornness as he did.

Vassilis had quickly made up for the lessons he had lost, thanks to the notes he had been lent by his new Greek friends, who in turn had borrowed those notes from their Italian classmates, who in turn had borrowed those notes from *me*, since I was notorious throughout school for my stubbornness in transcribing them all in fair copy in numbered and ordered notebooks, divided by subject, after each lesson. That's how I learned that Vassilis had studied from my notes during the entire school year, even though he was in a different section than me.

It was a revelation.

Suddenly I realized that I had been useful for something. To someone. Unbeknownst to me, I had indirectly helped a total stranger. It was an utterly bizarre and amazing discovery.

Vas, in turn, had not realized that I was the author of those notes until that day. Now that he knew, he would be grateful to me for a long, long time.

That episode was in some way the beginning of it all. The first flapping of wings of my own personal *butterfly effect*.

According to the chaos theory, a small change in the state of a nonlinear system can result in huge differences in a later state. For instance, a simple movement of molecules in the air generated by the flapping of the wings of a butterfly can cause a chain of events, even unleashing a hurricane on the other side of the world.

That discovery that day would move molecules which by strange and unknown ways would later change my life.

But I still could not imagine it. I was a year away from the final effect. One year away from the hurricane.

Matters of the Heart

It was time to go home.

The course in contactology was over and nothing more could provide me an excuse to stay in Vinci. All my classmates would, in any case, soon be leaving for various destinations within just a few days. Donatella invited me to her hometown in Sicily to spend the summer with her and her friends, and I came back home happy to have something to wait for.

In August, during my Sicilian stay, I met several of her friends who had visited her in Vinci. One of them attracted me immediately, as he was very open with me and full of affectionate attentions. I started fantasizing about a possible romance; but at the end of the holiday I faced the usual sad reality: I had no hope of having any kind of relationship with Donatella's friend, except for a simple friendship.

As I came home, my heart was filled with negative feelings: a mixture of frustration, desolation, and helplessness. I was realizing that those crises were following one another with increasing frequency. In high school, I had to deal with just a couple of such moments, whereas in Vinci they had intensified and multiplied, exponentially close to each other. Alarmingly.

Those peaks of despair, filled with streams of solitary tears, were by now an almost monthly occurrence, despite a climate of confidence and affection that I had never experienced before. Perhaps this was the reason: I had been welcomed so spontaneously and naturally at the optical school that it had nurtured the illusion of being able to have high hopes and had cultivated expectations that were unthinkable until then. Forbidden dreams. And the disappointment in seeing my failure was overwhelming. If I were not able to accomplish my romantic fantasies in such a welcoming and friendly environment, then I'd have no chance to succeed ever, as I would never find myself in such favorable conditions again.

In my hometown no one had ever approached me in such a disarming way as had happened in Vinci. Neither in the past nor in the future, I was adamant about that. My conviction strengthened whenever I came back home on the weekends and went out with my childhood friends. The faces we met while we were out for a walk or in pubs were always the same, those who had never taken me into account. The prospect of finding a boyfriend was simply ridiculous, close to zero.

Therefore, the failure at Vinci weighed on me as a huge, exaggeratedly heavy burden. True, there were still two years before the end of school, but by then I already knew pretty well all of my schoolmates. If nothing had happened during that first year, then it would not happen later on. I would have to get over it.

The following October, at the beginning of our second school year, Donatella and I moved to another apartment together, within walking distance of the institute, and were joined in our tiny new flat by a new female friend, Milena. She came from the region of Calabria, in Southern Italy, and had an outgoing nature, exuberant yet very sweet. What is more, she was extremely attentive to other people's needs—especially mine. For

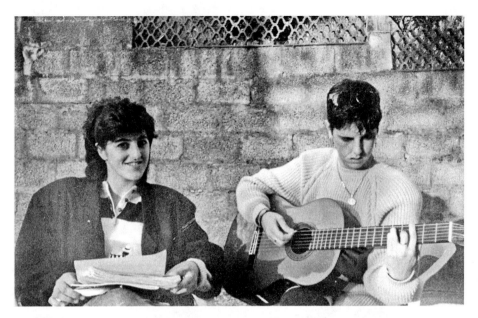

My friend Milena and I at Vinci, Spring 1990. Playing the guitar was one of my favorite hobbies from the time I was a teenager.

instance, she immediately noticed, even before Donatella, that I was a victim of the crush of the century.

In that period we used to hang out with the professors' assistants, who were almost our peers. We had met them during the summer course in contactology and now we related to them on very friendly terms. Donatella and I were especially close to one of them, Giampaolo, and the reason was obvious to everyone. The reason was me.

As a result, Milena felt a duty to do something about it. In order to help me in any way, she kept coming up with new and original pretexts to invite the unfortunate assistant to our place. Of course, I tried to camouflage my feelings as best as I could, but the truth was too obvious to be hidden.

We all hung out with Giampaolo throughout the winter and the following spring. My new flame used to come over to our place for lunch or dinner, although always hidden from prying eyes. After all he was a teacher, and it was not ethical for him to be seen hanging out with female students.

I knew right away that this story too was going to be filed under failure. Still, Milena, with tireless efforts, tried whatever she could to bring us closer. My diary testified to the day-by-day evolution of that new one-way, nonalternating romance: pages of joy following a little hint of affection towards me, mixed with pages of discouragement and disappointment due to ambiguous, sometimes indecipherable behavior.

My obsession with Giampaolo had literally switched my brain to overload mode. One day I was swearing eternal love to him, and the next I would hate him because he'd addressed just a few words to me. The well-known state of unrequited love. A classic, as far as I was concerned.

Same attempts. Same hopes. Same mistakes. Same rejections.

Then, at some point, everything changed.

One Face One Race

Towards the end of the second school year, Donatella, Milena and I had got very close to a Greek couple. Eléni and her boyfriend, Loukàs, were very nice, and often said that it had been easy for them to assimilate Italian customs because, after all, Italians and Greeks were, as they used to say in their language, "*mia faza mia raza*": that is, one face, one race. Similar in so many aspects, almost brothers. It was a very common saying in Greece. Soon, very soon I would understand the full meaning of that expression—in a matter of days.

The friendship with Eléni and Loukàs brought us to meet other members of the Greek community in Vinci, a diverse group of people we had never really got to know very well.

Until then, we knew very little about those Greek students. They were notorious for their infamous wild parties—filled with alcohol, loud music and traditional dances—but only a few lucky Italians were allowed to take part in them, usually roommates with some Greek guy who invited them accordingly.

At school, in class, they always sat in the back rows. Together, in close ranks like an army. After lessons they gathered in the main square, speaking in their language, and were rarely involved in our circles of friends.

As far as I was concerned, there had been only a few episodes where I could say that I crossed their world.

One was destined to remain in the collective memory, of both the Italians and Greeks in Vinci, as an unforgettable, hilarious anecdote. One day in class, during an enormously boring lesson, the professor just could not stop the buzz of conversation coming from the back row. The professor himself, however, caused the problem: he was extremely shy, insecure, and unable to keep the students' interest alive.

That day there was that constant noise coming from the back row. Exasperated, the professor called out a Greek boy's name and threw him out of class. However, within a few minutes the murmur was just as strong as before, and the teacher expelled another Greek student. But it was no use, there was still too much noise.

It was then that, red-faced, stammering, the professor uttered the words that would remain in the school's annals.

"All the Greek people, out!"

After an initial moment of confusion and disconcertment, at least 30 people stood up as one, snickering in amusement and disbelief, and left the room—emptying it almost completely.

From that day on their large group was renamed "the Greek people." So on and forever.

Aside from my meeting with Vassilis, who had made such an impression in my mind, before that spring in which we were introduced to the Greek community I remembered having exchanged a few words with another Greek guy. He was cute, but he wore an unlikely pair of old-style eyeglasses that covered his face almost completely. I would never have noticed him, as I had been indifferent to all his fellow Greek friends, were it not for an amusing, bizarre habit of his. When he arrived at school, while walking up the stairs that led to our class on the second floor, he sang. Always, every day, every time he entered the room. In a high voice.

Funny.

And he sang Italian songs, melodic ones, those I also used to listen to at that time.

Funny.

Once I asked him why he did not sing any Greek songs, and he replied that he much preferred Italian ones because when he sang them he felt "something inside."

Very funny.

That was my first encounter with Jorgos—Giorgio for the Italians— at the beginning of the second school year. Actually, I had no idea what his name was. Then, came June of that magic, unforgettable 1991.

June 25

May 23

In the afternoon Milena and I hung out in the square, to talk with the Greek guys. We're getting more and more friendly with them. I saw

Giampaolo for a moment, but did not even greet him. However, after dinner he stopped by our place. I was so happy. I missed him so much this evening. Why am I not coherent in my feelings? Then Milena went out, leaving us alone to talk until midnight. Felt good. Very good.

May 31

Today I started to cry and it seemed that I would never stop. I had the biggest hysterical crisis in recent times.

I'm tired of living. Seriously. More and more often I have to pretend to be happy in front of my parents and then I run to my room and cry, without them noticing so that they won't worry. But this time I did not manage to. This time I was exasperated.

There's nothing worthwhile in life. Nothing. I am tired of fighting against everyone; I can't do it anymore.

I don't think this time I'll get out of this crisis. Even now, after hours and hours, I keep crying in despair. I just can't stop the tears.

Mom realized that the very fact of not having a boyfriend weighs over me. And this makes me feel even worse. I feel humiliated.

And then ... there is the whole situation: day after day spent confronting myself and clashing with other people, the fear of their judgment, the inability to react aggressively to all this. I do not have a temper; I cannot face people's attacks. I can't even reciprocate those insistent, obnoxious looks. How can I go on like this with my head down, my eyes constantly pointed toward the ground? I'm close to collapse. Totally.

June 12

I came back to Vinci to study for my exams and attend the last lesson. Saw Giampaolo in the lab.

I can feel he is more detached than usual, and did not even talk to him. Who knows, perhaps he is in love for real, this time. Lucky him. But I must forget him, absolutely. Must keep him out of my head—but how can I?

June 13

After dinner we gathered in the square, singing and playing the guitar. There were lots of people, including many Greeks. Milena, Donatella and I are increasingly linked to them. Some are incredibly nice, but overall they are very sweet and affectionate. They are very friendly towards me and I don't know why. But I do not want to get involved with anyone, do I?

It feels so good to my heart being with them, as it helps me forget Giampaolo. There is a boy named Stratos who plays the guitar beautifully, so much better than me. And Jorgos sings very well, but I had already noticed that—how couldn't I? He's been singing all the way to the classroom, every day since the beginning of school! He always seems happy and carefree. We played many Italian songs, and then they played a few Greeks ones for us, melodic and poignant.

We enjoyed it all enormously. What a fantastic night!

June 14

Giampaolo stopped by in the afternoon, and we made a trip by car to Empoli.

I had a great desire to see him, but I immediately regretted it, because I had decided to ignore him. And until this evening I succeeded very well.

There was tension between us, and I almost didn't utter a single word. I must not give him such importance.

Tomorrow he is coming to our place for lunch, but I have decided that I will not be there.

June 15

At lunchtime I went out to study and sunbathe. All this because I did not want to meet Giampaolo. It's the first time I act like this, and I'm not feeling guilty about it. Of course he did not ask about me, but the girls told me he suggested we all make a trip to the sea tomorrow. I decided I'd go with them. Not seeing him hurts just me, and I'm not proving anything to anyone. It's all wrong.

We spent the evening playing mime with the Greeks. So much fun! I noticed a cute Greek lad but I don't even know his name ... tomorrow I'll check. Or rather, on Monday. Tomorrow I'm busy....

June 17

Just passed another exam! It went very well and I'm so excited! Saw Giampaolo outside the school but he did not pay much attention to me. However, all the teachers were there with him. Never mind.

Evening: Nikos (the cute one that struck me the other evening), Stratos, Jorgos, Vassilis and Loukàs came over to sing and play at our place.

I think Milena likes Stratos a lot, but I'm not sure. Will investigate.

They are all very nice and attentive towards me. I felt at the center of attention! It is such a beautiful and new sensation. During the evening Vassilis took me aside and asked some funny questions. He wanted to know who among us girls did not have a boyfriend.

Well ... what to think? He has got his own girlfriend in Perugia and I don't think he is investigating for himself. He is too honest a guy to do that. Milena says that perhaps he is scouting ahead for his best friend, Jorgos. Perhaps Jo is in love with Milena or Donatella. In fact, I've been thinking about that for some time.

The happiness of this evening is something I will always remember. I feel so good with my new friends!

June 20

Days all the same. As soon as I get out of school I spend the afternoon studying and after dinner I always meet our Greek friends at the main square. They are all very sweet and likeable: they even laugh at all my jokes! To think that I'm now such an irresistible joke-teller! But I can feel that they are sincere, and then they ask a lot of questions, and take an interest in me. I feel flattered, pampered, highly regarded. Finally someone is noticing me.

I seldom see Giampaolo these days, but I don't care. These new friendships are good for my heart and I hardly think about him.

Nikos and I have a nice friendship but nothing in particular. Never mind. This time, before falling back in the same situation as with Giampaolo, I'm going to think about it very very very very MUCH!

June 21

Last day of school! And the good news is that Milena is in love with Stratos.

I'm rooting for them; they deserve each other. Go Milena!

June 22

Studied all morning. Went to the pool with the Greek boys who threw me into the water twice! After dinner we all went to Florence.

Nikos: nothing in particular but I do not mind at all. Instead I talked quite a lot with Jorgos alone, while walking. He asked a lot of questions, and even asked if I would pay him a visit in his hometown of Corfu. It is a beautiful Greek island—who knows, I may think about it, I said. However, he was delighted, thrilled. And I was, too.

I kind of like Jorgos, he is always so funny and smiling. With those huge glasses, he makes me tender! But I don't want to make the mistake of falling in love again, now that I have almost succeeded in forgetting Giampaolo. I scarcely think about him now. Almost never.

Enough with suffering, ok? I'll never fall in love again. I swear!

June 23

What a day! FANTASTIC, but I want to keep my feet on the ground. I have to. Otherwise I'd start to fly, as usual, and if I fell I would hurt myself a lot. Quite a lot this time.

So: I studied all day (nothing fantastic there). After dinner we met the Greek boys at the main square and played our game of mimes, as usual.

At a certain point Jorgos showed up, looking very sad. I asked him if there was anything wrong, but he almost got angry. I did not pay much attention to him as the evening went by, but I was sorry to see that he was in such a low mood. It was very strange as he is usually so happy ...

He almost did not speak a single word throughout the evening. Then, at half past midnight, all the others went away, but I was not tired and Jorgos said he would stay there on the bench with me and talk for a bit. Well, that "bit" lasted until 4 in the morning!

It was amazing! First of all he explained that he was sad because nobody had told him that we would all meet that night, whereas he was very keen to be there since he felt so good being with us girls.

First small attack of heartache. Small, because he'd been too generic and certainly could not allude to me in particular. Still, while we were talking it seemed to me that I was living one of my daydreams, those that I used to get lost in when I was a child, every night before falling asleep. I heard myself saying things that I had repeated a million times in my head and I never thought I would say in real life to a real boy!

But let's move on slowly. I must explain exactly what happened so as to thoroughly analyze the night we spent together. I must not forget anything!

This evening Stratos came at our place to study with Milena, but of course our hope was that it would be a good chance for them to get together. Jorgos and I spoke a little about this, and at one point I asked him if he was in love with Milena, because I've always had this feeling.

He replied that it was not like that at all, but he imagined that I thought so. So I asked him if Donatella was the one he liked. He assured me that it was not even her that he was interested in....

My heart sank. Seriously, this time. I had the feeling he was trying to say something but could not manage it. Or did not have the courage.... But maybe it's just an impression, I thought, it must be that way—it's impossible he is referring to me. However, I did not ask him directly, I just would not be able to. The subject remained in the air ... underlined by his deep sigh and the words "Oh, Cristina..."

However, I told him that I had suspected this for a while, and that my suspicions were confirmed when the other night at our place Vassilis asked me those strange questions about which one of us had a boyfriend and which did not. Jorgos replied that Vas did it all on his own, he hadn't asked him to investigate. Soon after, however, he added: "And Vassilis asked you as well if you had a boyfriend, didn't he?" Sure, I replied. "And you said no, adding that you were not important, right?" Those were the exact words I had used with Vassilis: I was not important; no one would be interested in my relationship status on purpose.

Jorgos knew my answers, word for word! So I asked myself, and I'm still asking: why did he remember them so well? Who knows!

However, I explained that I answered like that because I never thought I could be of interest to anyone, I never had a boyfriend and would not even know where to start. He had to know the truth. And Jo told me he had a similar character to mine.

So, feigning indifference, I asked whether he had had girlfriends in the past and he confessed that he never had any. I could not believe it: my dream ... finding a boyfriend who has not had any girlfriend. The thing that made me suspicious is that he kept making those big sighs, followed by that enigmatic "Oh, Cristina..." suspended in the air ... and I just did not understand what he was trying to communicate. I mean, I imagined it, but couldn't believe it: I had to have a direct confirmation.

Eventually I got brave and asked him what all those sighs meant and ... at that very moment we saw Stratos coming out of our doorway, so I'll never know the answer!

I am so excited and confused. Back home I told Milena everything about my night, as well as Jorgos' sighs and ambiguous words, and she said it's definitely as I think it is.

But I don't want to rely too much on hopes, because otherwise I would be so badly disappointed! I so much wish it was like that, though. It would be awesome, amazing ... but impossible.

No, no. It is not conceivable. And yet I still have hope. But it cannot be. However ...

Well, as that Lucio Battisti song goes, we will only find out by living.

June 24

Morning, contactology test. Afternoon, at the pool with the Greeks. All but Jorgos. I really wanted him to be there but I certainly couldn't go and call him over....

I had not met him all day, and returned from the pool very much wanting to see him. And I did run up against him for a brief moment, just before dinner. He greeted me with a 32-tooth smile! So maybe it's true!

But no, I still can't believe it. Cannot be. A smile does not mean anything after all. He asked where I had been and with whom, and when I told him he was disappointed that nobody had invited him, again—but how could I?

Then in the evening we gathered again at our usual place. Three of us, including myself, had carried a guitar, and there were lots of people singing—Italians, Greeks, optics and optometry students.

Jorgos showed up almost immediately and sat behind me, on the back of the bench. So close that I could lean my back against his legs. At one point, while I was playing, I felt his hand on my shoulder!

But I did not give much importance to it. I am too scared of suffering. Actually, I was in a bit of a low mood during the evening since I didn't notice any particular attitude towards me on his part. I thought that perhaps I had been dreaming it all.

Then Milena called me aside and told me that throughout the evening Jo had been trying to put his hand on my shoulder but pulled back at the very last second. In the end, when he finally managed to, she and Donatella hugged each other!

At the end of the evening I went to bed a little sad and a little happy. I can't fool myself. It's impossible that this is really happening to me. It would be a dream.

But do dreams exist?

June 25 (the 25 surrounded by a big heart)

A HISTORICAL day. JORGOS AND I GOT TOGETHER!

I still don't believe this. It sounds unreal, unlikely, absurd, unbelievable, and miraculous.

First things first: this morning we had the English class test and Jorgos was there. I hoped he would be, because today I would leave for home and if he did not show up I would go without saying goodbye to him.

After school we invited him and Stratos to our apartment, and while I was packing my bags he came to my room to keep me company. I do not know how I managed to stay focused enough to pick up things and put them inside my suitcase. I was so nervous, and there was a bit of embarrassment in the air. I thought that if neither of us took the courage and spoke, we would never get to the point.

Then he told me that tonight he finally fell asleep at 5 in the morning. He could not sleep.

My heart stopped for a moment, but I did not ask him why. Too direct. Too much fear. Terror, I'd say. Then, when it came the time to bring my bags to the car, I couldn't find the keys. Jo had already mentioned, jokingly, that I would have a hard time finding them, but I didn't pay attention at first. So I got in the car to look for them and he followed me.

At one point he took the keys out of his pocket. I asked why he had hidden them and he replied that he did not want me to leave.

Tump! Another heartbeat lost forever. I thought I would pass out right then and there, but I decided I should feign indifference and look for some more clues. The shell of distrust I had built during all these years would not soften so easily.

We went back in the flat and I started saying goodbye to all of them when, in front of everyone, Jo asked to wait a little bit more. In a flash, all the others disappeared! I don't recall how it happened, the only thing I know is that one moment we were all together, and the next he and I were sitting in the kitchen, talking. Alone.

"Ok, if you want me to stay a little more at least you have to explain why the other night you always kept repeating 'Oh, Cristina.'"

"I hoped you'd get it."

"It can't be what I'm thinking."

"Why not?"

"Because it's absurd, inconceivable."

"No, it's not."

"Look…. I'm so happy but this is a total mess."

"Why?"

"Because I don't know what to say, what to do, where to start."

"To me, it's exactly the same. But if we feel for each other, if there is love, we can solve all problems."

"You don't understand…. I have a lot of insecurities, doubts, fears. You'd put yourself into trouble, real trouble…"

"I don't think so. I swear I can overcome any obstacle. I like you too much not to try."

"How long have you been feeling like this?"

"A few weeks, since I started to know you better. But I've always admired you. Then, in these last few days, I took courage and spoke to Stratos. The fact that he was interested in Milena helped me. I was suffering a lot and had to talk to someone. I could not sleep anymore because I kept thinking about you. All the time. I cannot study, cannot do anything. Last night, after we said goodbye to each other, I was on fire."

"Well…. I don't know what to say…. It seems incredible. I don't understand what you see in me. I have nothing to offer."

"Don't talk like that. You have a lot to give."

"I'm saying this for you, I want you to know what you are about to go through. You don't realize..."

"Let me decide what's best for me, will you?"

"But ... are you sure?"

"One-hundred-percent sure. One-thousand-percent. One-million-percent."

Then I leaned against him and Jo hugged me tight. He held my hands all the time.

Never in my wildest dreams could I have wished for such words. A scene I'd imagined a million times, in endless variations. But this time it was for real!

Well, it did happen! I still can't believe it. It seemed it was someone else living those moments, not me. Like watching a movie. A feeling I could not describe, even if I tried endlessly. Knowing that someone wants to touch me, hold me, kiss me ... is something I still find difficult to accept. We did not separate from the moment we first hugged each other.

It was an amazing feeling.

Jo took me to the car and there he gave me the first real kiss! I don't know if it was beautiful or not for him, but it was so sudden and heartfelt that I did not have the time to think about anything! All I know is that right afterwards Jo hugged me tight and told me he loved me. Me too, so much.

I can never thank him enough for what he has done to me. He doesn't know how important this day has been. Even if it all were to end tomorrow, I would still have experienced one day of absolute, total joy.

I came back home feeling a mixture of happiness, confusion, and worry. There are a million unanswered questions in my mind. Will I be able to give him what he wants? Will he still be so sweet and understanding tomorrow, the day after tomorrow, always? It is useless to torture myself like that. I must live this experience day by day.

This evening he called me and started the conversation with "Hello, my love..."

For the hundredth time, I thought it was all a dream. Even now, after hours thinking about it, I still cannot believe what is happening to me. Can one put up with a joy so devastating? Having a boyfriend who loves me, who thinks about me, who does not sleep because of me, is something unthinkable. But is this all really going on?

July 1

Back to Vinci. I was afraid of meeting him (because of the kiss, a fear that I've been carrying with me since a lifetime), but Jorgos just hugged me tight.

At one point we finally kissed and it was very sweet. I found out I do not have the problems that I thought I'd have, and all came so natural and beautiful. An unexpected surprise. To think that I tormented myself for years about this.

He loves me, and tells it to me all the time, in his own language.

S'agapò.

It seems a very sweet language to me.

But there is a problem. Jo's parents are not happy that he found himself an Italian girlfriend. His father is building a house for him and will never accept he moves away from Corfu. It is premature to think about these things, but if it were necessary I would follow him everywhere. I don't think I'll ever be happier than in these days. Never. Not even if I miraculously found another boyfriend. These feelings are and will always be priceless, irreplaceable, incomparable.

July 3

Today Jorgos was sad. After a while he told me that he called his parents and told them about me—the way I am, I mean. They were not happy. They wished a beautiful girlfriend for their son.

Isn't it amazing? Isn't it ironic? Isn't it cruel? Now that I finally found a boyfriend who does not care about my appearance, his parents do!

I cried in frustration. Despite everything, he still keeps telling me that he loves me so much and that I am beautiful to him! But what does he see in me? I don't know.

In one thing I was right. I would never live again those first, unknown and overwhelming emotions. Or rather, I would not feel them with the same, alarming intensity. I had fulfilled an impossible dream—*the* impossible dream. The father of all dreams, past, present and future. All of a sudden I was thrown into a wonderful world full of sensations that were amazing, unbelievable, unimaginable—a lot of adjectives, in fact, which I liberally scattered, page after page, in handfuls, during that magic July 1991.

Each moment of the day, each new event, was perceived as completely different from "before." At school, we entered hand in hand. Among friends, Jo held me close to him. All was new, unexplored, and magic. It was like being born to a new life, as if the previous twenty years had been archived within a few days.

No, in the future I would not experience such devastating feelings. Pure emotions, devoid of any shadow of doubt. A period of my life had ended, locked up with a bright red padlock. Red as heart, flower, and love, as the lexicon of any young girl demanded.

The moments of crisis that just a few weeks earlier had reached an alarming peak were now gone for good. Never again would I cry tears of loneliness and self-pity. No more. What I still could not imagine was that I would cry other kinds of tears in the future. Maybe I sensed it fleetingly. But the bad thoughts did not have much room in my mind during that first summer spent together with Jorgos. I was charged with an almost mystical fatalism: what will be will be. And the watchword of the day—of every day—was "live the moment."

Carpe diem.

The Long Hot Summer

That July was really intense. I had to undergo written and oral exams with a tiring frequency. I studied at night so as to spend every instant of the day with Jo. There were just a few days left before our separation for the summer holidays, and I would never miss a single moment of happiness.

Believe it or not, Nancy, I even started cooking for him, even though I did not even know where to start with it. I worked all morning on my very first culinary creation, thinking about how to present it, but when I finally brought my masterpiece to the dining table there was a moment of embarrassing silence.

"Uhm ... what is that supposed to be?"

"Veal carpaccio on a lettuce bed with parmesan cheese shavings, my love."

"You mean I have to eat *raw* meat?"

It became one of his favorite anecdotes. When Jo later told his Greek friends about it, they used to shiver at the thought: you know, in Greece the idea of eating raw meat is some sort of a sacrilege—cook your meat, and cook it well done! Jo did eat that carpaccio, but for months he paid me back by ironically reminding me about that succulent first meal I prepared him.

Men. How ungrateful.

Towards the end of July we had to say good-bye to each other: I would join my parents at the seaside, whereas he would go back to Greece with Vassilis and Ioanna.

The separation was not particularly traumatic: I had fantastic information to share with my whole family and was anxious to do it as soon as possible, as until that moment I had not told anyone the sensational news.

Except one person.

Early in July I had received an unexpected phone call.

"Hi, Cri, how are you?"

"Laura! I'm very, very good! But what a surprise!"

"I so much wanted to hear from you! I dreamt about you last night, you know? You whispered something in my ear, but I could not understand.

You know how dreams are—I have been thinking about this all day, and decided to give you a call. Is everything OK at your end?"

"Oh Laura, you'll make me cry. Wonderful, everything's going wonderfully. Actually, I have something to tell you, but you must keep it a secret. No one knows about it yet!"

Silence.

"Laura?"

Silence.

"Laura? Are you there?"

"I knew it. I knew it would happen at last. I was positive about that, Cri!"

"Now you are making me cry."

Long silence.

"Cri, I'm so happy—you can't understand how much. Do you believe me when I say that I always knew that this day would come?"

"Yes, Laura, I do. I believe you. You have always been there. I know that my sufferings were yours as well. And now, at last, I am happy. *One-hundred-percent*. Now I know what it means."

"You will tell me everything about it soon, will you?"

"Of course, Laura, we'll see each other at the beach. I'm coming over in a few days."

"Good. I'll wait for you then. And I won't tell anyone, don't worry."

"Thank you, my dear! So, see you soon."

"Cri?"

"Yes?"

"I love you."

"I know, Laura. I love you so much, too."

Tears, tears, tears. During the phone call, after the phone call—Another sensational discovery to be added to the wealth of emotions of those latest days. The sharing of absolute happiness caused more of the same—a whole lot of it! Would I be able to endure it? Was it possible to experience an overdose of happiness? I was starting to worry about it seriously.

My best friend had sensed from miles away that something had changed: were we really *that* close or was it just a lucky coincidence? I did not know, and I did not care. Life was beautiful, and was finally smiling. At me. Who had never managed to smile at her.

That summer away from Jorgos seemed endless. After the first few days of euphoria when I got back home, time began to mysteriously slow down, and the days seemed to drag on and on. I told the great news to my parents, who reacted enthusiastically. I had not doubted that they would: they had finally achieved one of their greatest goals—to see me happy. *One-hundred-percent* happy.

They did not even bat an eyelid when I told them that Jo was Greek. To them, it did not matter. They were just very curious to meet him, perhaps because of his nationality but more likely to understand who this person was who had taken me away from the brink of an insignificant life.

Even my sisters had greeted the news enthusiastically, even though each of them did so in a manner appropriate to her own character. Tiziana reacted with her typical exuberance—with a hug that could even choke me, as far as I knew. Rossella—who in the meantime had become the mother of a beautiful little girl and was expecting her second child—gave me one of her sweetest and most seraphic smiles. One of those smiles that meant everything to me.

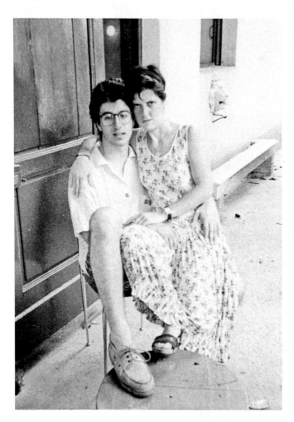

In those early days of separation, I regularly received phone calls, more and more often full of phrases such as "I miss you" and "I can't live without you."

Jo had finally left for Greece, and Vassilis told me, during a hilarious phone conversation, that in the cabin of the ship that was taking them to Corfu, Jorgos had been talking in his sleep all night, repeating my name now and again. From then on, time dilated more and more. Each day away from him seemed like a week, and despite exchanging long-distance calls at regular intervals, each of us confessed to the other that it looked like the summer would never end.

June 1991. My first days in Vinci with Jorgos, both looking very, very happy.

Jo continued to play

the role of the perfect boyfriend. On the phone he was very sweet and always seemed to guess the most critical moments of the day, as his calls came at just the right moment, almost as if he were able to read my thoughts. He even sent a package with a small gift and flowers. Seven red roses. A strange number, which in retrospect, many years later, I understood as prophetic.

There was only one small detail that caused me a little inner torment. From Corfu came not-so-reassuring news regarding his parents. They were puzzled by the fact that I was a foreigner, and even more so after seeing some pictures of us together. They realized that it would not be easy to introduce me into their family. My physical defect would be the talk of the town, a whole community of family and friends. Soon I would find out the hard way how strong the concept of "family" is in Greece.

Jorgos's parents had sensed from the beginning that we would be judged by all and put under a huge magnifying glass. For this reason they were warning their only male offspring. Jorgos had to have understood it from the early stages of our relationship. My new fiancé was still reasoning with the heart not the mind, and he told me to stop worrying as everything would be all right in the end. I, with all the baggage of relationship difficulties that I carried with me, had immediately realized that this would be a big issue in our love story. And even though I tried to think positively I felt there was still a shadow to darken my *one-hundred-percent* happiness.

At the end of that summer my family received an unbelievably high phone bill: one million and six hundred thousand *lire*. Pure madness. And yet Jo beat me: his phone bill was twice as much as ours. By the end of August we were phoning each other even four times a day. It was especially Jo who made surprise calls that every time intoxicated me with newfound happiness and assured me of his unconditional love. Always the right call at the right time. Given my insecure character, I needed them as I needed lifeblood.

If a single day had passed without the confirmation of his feelings, I would have gone into crisis. My inner fragility rose with the passing of time. I would never attain total serenity because, quite simply, I could not.

I was constantly assailed by doubts, questions, and hesitations. Would I be able to prevail over the judgment of Jo's relatives? Would he love me as much forever? Or would he find some other girl who could make him even happier?

These doubts—I would drag them along over the years. I have never been able to deal with our relationship calmly. I always had the feeling of living that experience while hanging by a thread, strong but fragile at the same time.

A precarious balance. And unstable, too.

Jo made me the ultimate gift of that endless summer. He managed to come to Italy two weeks ahead of schedule. He wanted to surprise me, but finally he could not keep it a secret. In one of his numerous phone calls in August, he announced his arrival on September 8. For the occasion, he put back onto the road a very old Renault 5 that he had bought for a song.

That summer, because of him, I decided not to act in a play we used to put on every year with friends of the parish. I've always loved acting. It may seem strange, but despite the fact that the syndrome does not allow normal facial expressions, which are essential for stage plays, my acting always impressed the audience. A real mystery, but enjoyable. Giving up the annual play did not cause me any particular sadness: I disappointed a few friends, but this year my attention was focused exclusively on the arrival of my beloved Jo, and nothing else.

When the day finally came, the integration of Jorgos in my family and among my friends was immediate.

My father got on right away with that nice and friendly lad, who was the model of the son that never came into our family. My mother adored him for the simple reason that he was the sole and irreplaceable cause of my happiness. And my sisters welcomed him with open arms, and above all, gave him a new pair of eyeglasses to replace those huge and clumsy ones that I had been so touched by in the past.

In a few short days Jorgos had found a new family, new friends, a new house, and shiny gold metal frames waiting for him.

A good start to our new life together.

Islands

The intention was to leave almost immediately for the Island of Elba, in the Tyrrhenian Sea, the largest island of the Tuscan archipelago, where my parents owned a small apartment. We had planned to spend a few days together at the sea before diving headlong into the school year that would follow.

On that island, Laura had told me that she had had her first sexual experience with her new boyfriend, Gianni, early that summer. At last she found the peace she was looking for in this new relationship; she told me she was experiencing her first important love story, the one that would surely blossom into a solid and happy marriage. It might have sounded like a rash prediction, but after meeting Gianni during the summer I no longer had any doubts: Laura was serious about it. She had found her soul mate, the other half of the Platonic myth, and it filled me with joy—as much as to know that, for both of us, that year was magical and unrepeatable.

Of course I had already introduced Jorgos to Laura and Gianni, and we had dinner together on the first night of his arrival in Italy. They were the two people to whom I felt closest, apart from my family, and it was mandatory that they be the first to meet the protagonist of my new life as a formerly single woman. I wanted to know their opinion. And, conversely, I wanted to know how Jo would judge them.

We had a great time together, as if Laura and Gianni had known Jo for years: an old friend who had finally come back into our lives.

At the end of Jorgos's first day in Italy, which had been full of intense emotions, I wrote in the diary: "It was one of the most beautiful days of my life."

And it was true.

My father had bought a flat in the village of Porto Azzurro, on the western coast of Elba, the previous year, and the accommodation was perfect for the short pre-school holiday Jorgos and I had envisioned.

Those days were just perfect.

In that small apartment, I found myself playing the role of the hardworking wife who prepared lunch and dinner for her adored husband, an experience that only a few months before I never thought to live. I was plunged back into a bubble of happiness mixed with a sense of unreality, completely enraptured by all these novelties.

It had been raining all the time, but we did not care. We were almost always at home, exchanging tenderness interspersed with some moment of study for the exams that we would have to face in Vinci.

Then, the inevitable: in those magical days, it was natural for it to happen.

Our first time.

We came to it in a completely spontaneous way, without any embarrassment, through a path of infinite sweetness. For both of us it was the first time ever, and this made us free from any troublesome and unpleasant comparison. We were accomplices, sweethearts, and lovers. It was all new and wonderful for both of us, in the same way.

From that point on, I always had a special relationship with islands, even though I could not yet imagine that.

Corfu, where Jorgos lived, was an island.

Rhodes would be another important milestone in our history.

Cephalonia, Ithaca, Zakynthos, we would visit them again and again over the years.

And then, one day still far away, we discovered Paxos together—yet another small, unknown island—which would forever mark our future.

As soon as we arrived in Vinci, before we began the final school year, we had a look around to find an apartment to move into together. It so happened that a flat was available, next to the house where Vassilis and his girlfriend Ioanna lived. In the meantime she had decided to leave her studies in Perugia and had enrolled at the IRSOO herself.

Both our families had approved our cohabitation, though with some reservations, and there were the typical recommendations by anxious parents, as understandable as they are useless. Our new life under the same roof worked well, despite some disagreements, which, however, I considered as normal for a newly engaged couple.

Jorgos often went out with his Greek friends in the evening, and I stayed home waiting for him. Sometimes until late at night. When this happened, I would visit Ioanna, and we had long talks, comparing our relationships. She, too, felt lonely whenever Vassilis went out with Jo and the others, and we consoled each other, trying not to sound too possessive towards our boyfriends.

I learned very quickly that the men had different needs from us girls, the eternal romantics. Ioanna and I would always want to stay glued to them, but it certainly was not the other way round. It was quite clear by now. I would have to absorb, assimilate, digest this concept as soon as possible, but it was not easy. I thought of myself as still too much in debt to life as a couple. I still had to recover what I had lost on the way over the years. And so I suffered—moderately, but consistently—every time Jo went out. We also argued on several occasions because of this. Every time I came out of it with a broken heart: I hated fighting over some nonsense, but the nonsense was stronger than me.

One day we had a more heated argument than usual. The reason, always the same. I was aware of stressing him too much. Finally, after tears and tears, I apologized and promised to change. It would take some time for me to improve and weaken the possessiveness that characterized me. But slowly I would succeed.

I could not risk losing Jo for a reason so ridiculous.

It was unthinkable. Unimaginable.

The next morning, when I woke up, Jo behaved in a strange way and asked strange questions. He wanted to draw my attention to a small piece of paper that he had left next to my pillow. In perfect handwriting—although littered with small spelling errors—and in a bright red ink, Jo had written me the most beautiful love letter I had ever received:

My love.

It is 2.10, and I still cann not sleep. So I found the chance to write this little letter to you.

I want to tell you I lov you so much more now since all the time we've been together (from Junne so far).

Cristina I really now understand what a treasure I hold in my hands. The last few days I discovered the inner world of the girl who I hope will make me happy for life.

The invitation that I made to come to Greece was not by accident. I want my parents know you as soon as possible. They must also understand what a diamond God gave me (and I thank Him very much).

My love you must know that any problem you have is also mine. I'll help you with all the strength I have and if sometimes I get angery not because I'm bad but a little selfish.

And excuse me if I have hurt you. I sweer I won't be doing that again.

I love you infinitely
"O Jorgakis sou" (Your little Jorgos)

December came, and with it my first birthday as an engaged woman. Another "first" to be added to the many already experienced in the last few months.

My *little Jorgos* escorted me home whenever I had to return, such as for the birth of my second nephew, Samuele, in September of that year. On the few occasions when he was not coming with me, Jorgos always reached me on the phone, reminding me that it made no sense for him to just stay in our apartment without me.

In one of these periods of separation, I had to spend about a week at home with my parents. After four days I saw him enter the front door, casually humming an Italian song.

As if he had just walked up from downstairs to see me.

As if he hadn't just driven one hundred miles in his beat-up Renault.

As if surprises like that were his daily bread.

For a full minute I was speechless. Then we hugged each other strongly and blah, blah.

Jo was like that: he always managed to surprise me. How could I not worship Him with all my heart? At times like that, I was convinced that nothing would stop us—nothing and no one in the world.

But, unfortunately, I was wrong.

Christmas in Greece

We both had made the decision.

It was especially Jorgos who wanted it: for the Christmas holidays we would leave together for Greece and I would finally meet his parents. It was a moment I had feared for months now, but it had to be faced. For better or worse, they would have to meet me, and accept my place in their son's life.

I admired Jorgos's courage. Even though he knew what was waiting for him, he was moving forward, without hesitation. He really wanted to fight for our relationship, knowing that his parents would never agree to it, but he was hoping for a change as soon as they got to know me. He was sure, he said, that if they realized what a treasure I had inside of me, they would not make any further objection to our relationship.

He could see that treasure and did not accept it would not be visible to others. And so he fought, tenaciously, against everyone's advice. I had to support him, if only for the unwavering confidence that he had placed in our relationship.

We left with Vassilis and Ioanna, our closest friends and the accomplices participating in our mad mission. Their attendance at the first meeting with my new in-laws was essential, as they somehow distracted the attention that weighed on me—or at least, I felt calmer because of them.

I already knew some Greek words, but nothing fancy, just simple greetings and little more: it would have been impossible to have an elaborate conversation with Jorgos's parents. But luckily there were Ioanna and Vas who, throughout the dinner, helped to alleviate a situation that would otherwise have been quite problematic. And embarrassing. I would never be able to thank them enough. That evening they tried to involve me all the time, and even though I understood very little of their words in Greek, I guessed they were talking about me—of how sweet-smart-funny-cute-formidable I was.

They were priceless. The best friends one could ever ask for.

Jo's parents were extremely friendly and affectionate. If they had some hesitations when they finally saw me, they managed to hide them perfectly. His father looked very much like his son. He smoked a pipe, which instantly intrigued me, and was bursting with affection from every pore. I felt an instinctive sympathy for him right away, whereas I still had some reservations about my mother-in-law. But I was sure it was only a matter of time. Anyway, it is well known that mothers-in-law are always the painful part of a love affair, overprotective as they always are towards their offspring. In any case, the meeting seemed to have been positive. The parents were both intelligent and educated. I was confident that they would not object to our relationship, and would leave their son free to decide what he wanted to do with his life.

After a few days we all went together to Thessaloniki, to spend Christmas with Jo's sister and her husband. In capital letters on a huge mirror at the entrance of Natalie's flat, a line had been written for me: "*Welcome Cristina.*" I was moved. It was really kind and thoughtful of her.

Her husband made a very good impression on me. Angelos was a huge guy, six feet tall and over two hundred pounds of sympathy and smiles. After just a few days we were very close, always laughing and joking in a mixture of Greek and English that only the two of us understood. A very nice person, the kind you would hug from morning to evening.

In short, I was happy.

I had received a warm welcome from everyone, and Jo's parents kept congratulating me on how smart I was and quick to learn more Greek words each day. In fact, it was a great effort to speak in their language, but I noticed that I could figure out a good part of their conversations. The Greek language was harmonious and sweet to my ears. Until then, I had learned only romantic words, what Jo always said in moments of intimacy.

Agàpi mou, my love.

Latrìa mou, my darling.

Glikià mou, my sweet.

But thanks to Jo's friends, in Vinci I soon learned the more sordid four-letter words as well, and when in those days in Thessaloniki I mistakenly came out with one of them, general hilarity ensued.

I felt just fine. There would not be any of the problems that we had imagined.

It all would work out perfectly.

We stayed at Angelos and Natalie's place until our departure, at the beginning of January. We went back to Vinci, to our nest, serene, peaceful and more in love than ever.

Then, on January 12, cruel hands shook the magical crystal ball in which we lived. And came the storm.

All in the Family

Jorgos received a call and came back into the room with tears in his eyes. I had never seen him cry before and never saw him do so again. He had spoken at length with his father, who had told him about the scandalized reactions of the relatives and friends we had met during my stay in Greece.

During our stay there, we had also attended a family friend's wedding, and I was introduced there to a lot of people. Apparently, they had all had a terrible impression of my physical appearance. More or less, they were all shocked and horrified by the fact that Jo had a relationship with someone *like me*.

If I had still been a naive little girl I would ask, what does *like me* mean?

But unfortunately, I knew exactly what they were referring to: relatives and friends did not accept that one could feel affection, even love, for somebody who could not even manage overt facial expressions.

Someone with a crooked face.

A disaster.

A monster.

Some of them had not slept all night; others had not shown up at work because of grief. A whole community devastated. Since I still could not understand what an important role the concept of "family" had in the Hellenic culture, I was left stunned. In my private experience, cousins and uncles never had the right to intervene in any personal, family matter, and I could not imagine how Jo's parents might be so influenced by outsiders' opinions.

But I soon learned that in Greece family is sacred. It is intended as a single body, which includes generations of kin, up to third-degree cousins, at least. And each member of the clan must definitely take into account what the rest of the group thinks about any matter, because the family is everything, and you cannot disappoint any expectations.

It would be a sacrilege. Especially if you are the first-born male and you bring your grandfather's name, and therefore your first son will carry the name of your father. A rather serious matter, the heritage of an ancient tradition, difficult to oppose.

With my arrival, I had disrupted the communal harmony and broken all the rules of the right-thinking society. I represented an anomaly in the system, and as such I should disappear as soon as possible. Jo would have to start from scratch and get back on track.

He deserved better. He was destined for great things. He could not waste all his infinite potential with a being *like me* next to him.

Jorgos was crying and I did not know how to console him. To tell you the truth, Nancy, I did not even know how to comfort myself. What would happen now? Was it all over? Should I simply understand and step aside?

Jo had no answers to give me. I collapsed in a state of utter depression. After a long, painful discussion, we decided to wait for a few days. In any case we could not leave the apartment like that—on the spot. One of us would have to find a way of moving forward.

But in what state of mind?

No. No, no, no, no, no, no.

We could not. Not right away.

At the end of that tragic day we reached a compromise: we would be together until July, at the end of school. Meanwhile, Jorgos would have the time to think it over and choose what to do with his life. Everyone had warned him—his parents, his sister, other relatives. Jo would have to choose on its own, but he had to be careful and take into account future suffering, because of me.

And so, Jorgos had to decide what to do with me within a few months. At that point, I could only hope for a miracle.

The next few days were sad and forlorn. We were both devoid of any energy, exhausted and apathetic. I was trying to appear lively in front of him, but as soon as I found a moment alone I burst out crying bitter, help-less tears. I just had to be patient and wait.

Laura called, instinctively realizing as always what a defining moment in my life this was. I could not explain how she managed to phone when-ever I needed someone to talk to, but she always seemed to know it. I was desperate. I told her what had happened and she, with her unshakable optimism, played down the whole thing and reassured me by saying it would be resolved soon. It could not go any other way. I just had to be quiet, and everything would fix itself.

That phone call helped me a lot. From that day on, a slow recovery began for us both—a new beginning, which would help us to decide, just a few weeks later, that no one could separate us.

Jo said that he loved me too much to give up so easily, and he would fight for me. Always.

It was a fortune.

I was not yet ready to deprive myself of the relationship that had cat-apulted me into the wonderful world of normal people. I had confessed in June to my diary that just one day, one day of total happiness, would be sufficient for me to die happy. More or less, that was the sense of that entry.

But now everything had changed. Now that I had tasted what it meant to live life as a couple, it would have been a huge blow to go back to the daily routine, a combination of studio-home-work that I would never be happy living.

I could not tolerate it anymore.

A few months of absolute joy—of walking hand in hand, cuddles and caresses and kisses—would not be enough for me. I wanted to prolong the idyll for as long as possible, but that did not depend only on me. Miraculously, during those weeks Jo fell in love, seriously in love. He even started to tell me about the house his father was building and that we would decorate together, once it was ready.

I tried to keep my feet on the ground, but he always managed to drag me along, into those wonderful daydreams. I would not have any difficulty in following Jo to Corfu for good and starting a new life there. Nor would my parents ever prevent me: they loved me too much to deny me a future with him. I knew they would suffer because of the distance between us, but it would be an acceptable sacrifice, as long as they knew that their beloved daughter was finally happy.

For the Easter holidays Jorgos returned to Greece, this time without me. He promised that he would speak at length with his father, and he wasted no time doing so. The day after his arrival in Corfu, I received an excited phone call: his dad had realized how much he loved me and did not pose any objection to our relationship. Jo also told of another detail that served to dispel any doubt or suspicion in my mind: his mother placed three new photos in plain sight in their house's main lounge—pictures of me and Jo embracing, taken on the day that we become engaged.

That strategically located position in the lounge was a clear sign: our relationship had been approved and made official. It would be clear to all those who entered their home. Which, from that day, had become mine too.

That April, when Jo called me, excited about the positive reaction of his parents to our union, I was helping Rossella in the preparations for the opening of our own opticians' shop. I would not be working full time in there, though. From that summer a going to and coming from Greece would begin that would last for many years.

The first summer I spent in Corfu, along with Jorgos and his relatives, was just beautiful. His parents welcomed me like a member of the family who had been far away for too long. I was beginning to get by with the language, but my knowledge of Greek would never be strong enough—or at least, it was not on my first long stay in Greece.

One night, when Jo suffered terrible stomach pain due to a virus, I realized the hard way how inadequate and out of place I still was in that foreign country. At the critical moment when Jorgos was about to throw up, his mother ran to her bed and held his forehead with a wet cloth. In the meantime, she was shouting a word I did not know yet.

"*To lechàni! To lechàni!*"

"Oh my God ... what do you mean??? *Tì* ... ???"

"*To lechàni! To* LECHÀNI*!*"

"Damn it, I don't understand ... *dèn katalavèno...*"

"*To* LECHÀNI*! Pàre to* LECHÀNI*!*"

That embarrassing situation would have lasted for who knows how long, with Jo's mother yelling—more and more distressed—that damn word. And I would still continue to not understand. But how could I? Her shouting didn't make it any clearer. No, not really. It certainly did not help. It was only able to arouse in me a sense of helplessness that I would drag around for a long time afterwards.

In that situation I was proving totally useless, inadequate, unsuitable. Probably that woman was desperately regretting the fact that I was not Greek, and maybe she even hated me at that very moment—no, not maybe, she definitely did. While all these thoughts crossed my mind in the space of a nanosecond, with a whisper, as if by magic, Jo found the strength to help me and relieve me from an embarrassment bordering on parody.

"Cri ... a bucket..."

Sure! That was it! How silly of me!

What else would she ask for in a situation like that? Jo was sick and about to throw up and it did not occur to me that a damn bucket would be needed so as not to soil the bed. I ran in search of the now unforgettable *lechàni*, but I was sure that I would not find it in time. I could never be so lucky. Then, as fate would have it, his father showed up from around the corner with the object of my desires in hand: he had just saved me from a disastrous epilogue. And so it was that, hugging him, I spoke a sentence that I was certain of. As least that one I knew.

"Thank you, thank you very much. *Efharistò, efharistò polì.*"

That embarrassing episode aside, the summer was over in a flash, including trips to the beach and evenings around the house. Now I even liked going to the disco: the miracle of the union between two people in love.

So many things had changed in my life. In those days Laura and Gianni paid us a visit and going out together, all four of us, made our holiday unforgettable. I remember that one day, caught by the enthusiasm of the moment, Jo asked me when our best Italian friends would get married. I replied that it would take at least two or three years.

"Then we'll get married first!"

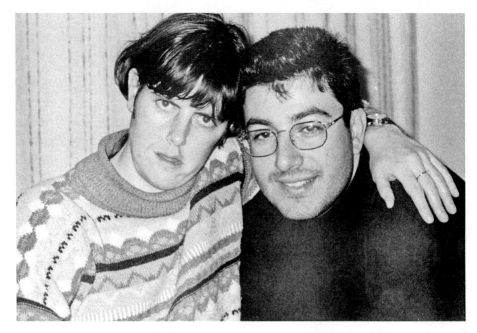

Winter 1994. Jorgos and I in Rhodes, where he was serving in the army. Those months were the most magical period of our relationship.

A phrase that made me happy, ecstatic.

I could not have wished for a more exciting situation than that. Jo was finally happy, and I was with the people to whom I felt closest. I had spent all my summer holidays with Laura and our families in the past—all of them, since kindergarten. It was a kind of tradition that should never stop. As it always had been, and as it always should be.

But, that would be my last holiday with Laura.

Nancy

That fall, upon returning to Italy, there were no postholiday dramas waiting for me, no new hysterical reaction from the relatives. Everything was going smoothly, and Jo seemed quiet from that point of view. In any case, I knew that that little black hole would always be present, even if not directly visible. A black hole that always had to be kept in check, or else some day it might devour the two of us. It was mainly for this reason that I decided to look for someone who might somehow improve my aesthetic condition. So many years had passed after the first, unnecessary surgery that I had undergone so full of hope. It was time to figure out if science had made any progress in dealing with the syndrome.

A cosmetic surgeon advised us to go to the town of Nancy, in France, and submit my case to the attention of the head of the maxillofacial department at the local hospital. We were told that he was renowned, and that he had solved all kinds of clinical cases in the past. It was time for me and my family to start down a new, untrodden path: looking for a solution to the syndrome abroad.

In October we all left for France, including Jorgos, for a check-up in the city that inspired me to give you this name, my dear Nancy. There, I was hospitalized for three days and turned inside out like a sock.

In a moment, I was transported back into the past by an invisible time machine: many years earlier, in another hospital, in another city. Suddenly I found the same sensors, the same electrodes, the same needles planted in any part of the body—always the same, even after years. Always painful and unnecessarily annoying. My body was littered with medical devices, again, looking for a breath of life in my facial muscles.

And I tried to bear all of it stoically, again, like the good girl that I had been in the past.

Finally, the professor told us that he could do something. He would pull a nerve from my temple, and connect it to the cheek through strips of synthetic fibers, which would also support the whole muscular structure. More or less.

I do not remember the exact procedure, but it was something like this: a new technique, never heard of before.

The surgery would not create new scars, this time. The professor would operate by reopening old wounds, not creating new ones. Or rather, there would indeed be a new one, but almost invisible, hidden behind the ear.

Eager as we were for solutions that would be easy and not too elaborate, what the doctor promised seemed wonderful to us: it would not be a real nerve transplant, but it would come very close. Even though the professor did not guarantee the surgery would be successful, it was well worth trying.

And so, after a few months, we set out for Nancy, full of new hopes, blinded by new daydreams. I was strongly hoping to be able to achieve some results, just to show Jo and his parents that I was committed to improving my appearance, that I was trying really hard to do something about it.

In fact I found it extremely difficult to have to deal with more surgery, which this time would be carried out under general anesthesia, an experience that I had never undergone, and that bothered me a bit. I was worried that something might go wrong, and I would never wake up. That would have been a shame. A real nuisance—now that I'd found the will to live that had been missing for so many years.

It was an absurd phobia, I was well aware of that. But I had every right to have some hesitation about it, don't you think? In the end it was my life. Mine, and no one else's.

The operation went smoothly.

And along with it came the expected results as well.

As I said, Nancy, when I woke up there was my mother holding my hand. She told me that everything had gone well. Between one postoperative nap and another, I also glimpsed Jorgos, standing at the foot of the bed and smiling at me but looking a bit worried.

A few days later we all went back home. The recovery was pretty fast, and since I had not been pierced with incisions inside the cheek, I was able to eat normally almost at once. Even the pain was moderate.

In the diary I reminded myself how much worse the 1985 operation had been in comparison. I wrote that I was satisfied with the results: for a few weeks I could finally feel the muscle responsible for smiling, I could move it and stretch it in the right direction.

I was thrilled, of course.

I remember that the first night after the great discovery I just could not sleep, because every now and then I would try to make it work: now that the muscle had been activated, I was scared to death that it would quickly get tired. Whereas I had to show a beautiful smile, the next morning, when Jorgos would come visit me at the hospital.

I trained for this moment all night, you know?

And I succeeded, to the delight of both of us.

Unfortunately, as I feared, after some time the little muscle's activity began to fade. I had been

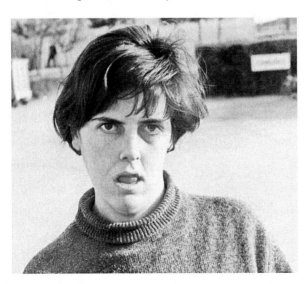

Winter 1992. A few days before leaving for Nancy, where I would undergo a major surgery.

recommended some physiotherapy to train it, but despite all my efforts, I could feel it was giving up. It was a great feeling to finally feel it alive and vibrant, but soon I had to realize that it was only a brief, unique interlude. And unrepeatable. Just two weeks after surgery, despite the daily exercises to try to stimulate the muscle, it was all over.

Zeroed. Reset. Rewind.

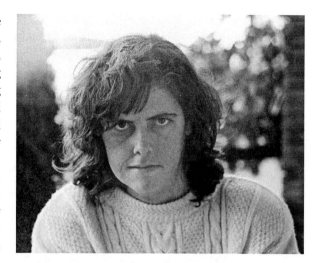

March 1993. The smile I had always wished finally manifested itself after the Nancy surgery only to gradually disappear a few weeks later.

We were back to square one: I, my parents, Jo. All of us. The right side of my face was once again still, as it had always been in the past.

After all these years, I still perceive that brief period when I tasted a bit of "normalcy" as a mystical event, almost unreal. Sometimes I doubt my memories, and I think I imagined it all. Is it possible that for a few days I was able to smile? I always tend to shake my head and say that no, it really seems absurd.

But I have evidence of it, Nancy: I had a picture taken of my face, as soon as I got back home. A snapshot that portrayed me with my lips closed, forming a smile. A sweet smile, symmetrical, perfect.

Around me, a soft glow from the late afternoon. A sort of luminous aura that over the years I've interpreted in a very personal way. I am convinced that it was supernatural. That it sprang from that smile that I had desired so much. A smile I had been waiting for so many, many, many years. A smile unique and unequaled. Mine.

Little by Little

After my surgery, Jorgos returned to Greece, full of new hope, which I tried to restrain, well aware that the results of the operation were only temporary, and that they would never manifest again.

I was back to work at the shop almost immediately. I loved that daily activity, as it made the days away from Jo seem shorter, as they came and went faster. Furthermore, I loved everything about my new job.

Very often customers came in and showed a little hesitancy in being received by me. Maybe because I seemed young or "inexperienced." But I sensed that there was also another reason. For many it was inconceivable that behind that expressionless face, so weird, there was a person capable of doing that job, or any other one for that matter. But I was not put off by their hasty judgments. I guessed at first what they were thinking, and I would prove them wrong. In fact, most of the time they left transformed, convinced that they had been assisted by a caring, professionally prepared, and, above all, very, very nice person.

If there is one thing I have always cared much about, it is the study of human psychology. My main goal, to my customers, could be summed up in one word: Empathy. Back then I did not know how to name this work of introspection. I found the exact word a few years ago.

Empathy. It seems a perfect term to me, harmonious and beautiful. It comes from the Greek, incidentally: "To enter the *pathos*." Digging in the soul, in feelings. Share them and experience others' emotions. A complete word that has always been the key to my way of relating to people from then onward.

At that time, I felt more self-assured just by the fact of having a boyfriend. I had proof that someone could love a specimen like me, with all my flaws, outer and inner. I was worth something, after all. I was still very far from reaching a manifested swagger, as I was still haunted by a million insecurities. However, working in the shop day after day gave me more confidence. I could be acceptable in other people's eyes, even friendly and jovial.

Of course, any daily confrontation with the next customer was like a challenge that renewed itself time after time. Sometimes I had to deal with people so obtuse that I just had to give up. Some customers did not even look me in the eyes and pretended I did not exist. As if that "Good morning, can I help you?" had been uttered by an alien.

Same old story.

In those cases I did not have any chance of succeeding. I sensed by myself when the challenge was too difficult, and I raised the white flag. I walked away and called my sister.

"Rossella, the lady is looking for you."

A defeat, that is true. But the next attempt would be better, I was sure. I had proof of it every day.

Sometimes I think that without my job I would not have developed the experience that today I think I have in dealing with people, and the capacity to understand how to interact with a new acquaintance—whether to listen to the other person with patience, to respond with determination, to joke together, or to console sympathetically.

Empathy. The most beautiful word I know.

I spent the spring of 1993 almost entirely in Corfu.

It was the first time I had stayed in Greece for so many months in a row. After all, if that was to be my future home, I should introduce myself in some way in their community. *The* community.

Imposing my presence next to Jorgos sometimes was complicated. One day at the supermarket where his family used to buy groceries, a cute young cashier asked him a question—a naive one, which nevertheless hurt me a lot.

"*Kalimèra, Jorgos. Pea ennui I copula aft? Mìa csadèlfi sou?*" (Good morning Jorgos, who is this girl, a cousin of yours?) No one thought that I could be his girlfriend. That was unacceptable.

Unfortunately, during my stay things were going from bad to worse. I realized that Jorgos had become impatient, apathetic, and distant. I did not know if the lack of results from my surgery played a part in that, but I had a strong suspicion that it did. After all, I could not work miracles.

The usual sense of helplessness, again.

I tried to take part in family life, lent a hand in his father's small clothing industry, but there was nothing to be done. Nothing worked. I saw Jorgos drift away from me and his love diminish day by day.

He was letting go, and he wallowed in some excesses I had never fully accepted. For one thing, he gained a lot of weight. Bad sign: he did not listen to my advice, or simply did not care anymore.

Towards the end of May I went back home feeling defeated, disappointed and scared. In the last few days we had argued all the time, and when the time for my departure came I felt a total indifference from him. I was aware of being back on the edge.

A few days after my return to Italy, following a few more and more insistent phone calls in which I demanded some concrete answers on his part, I received a fax at the shop. I remember very well the arrival of that paper that made my blood freeze. I was with was a former high school friend who was telling me she had escaped a terrible event. The day before she had been in Florence, near Via Georgofili, when a bomb had exploded, killing five people, including a newborn baby and a nine-year-old girl. It

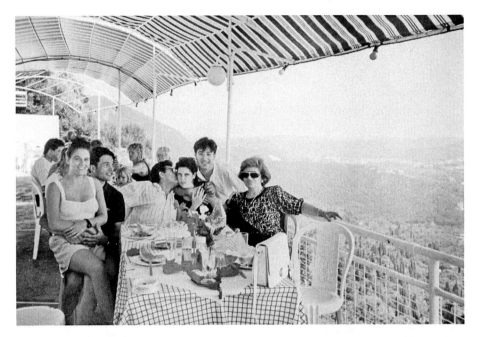

Summer 1992. On the isle of Corfu. With Laura and Gianni (on the left), Jorgos and his parents (his father is kissing me on the cheek).

later became known that the Mafia had put the bomb there; a few more bombings would follow that summer, putting our country in turmoil.

I was listening in disbelief to her chilling recollection of the event, when the phone rang, giving off the monotonous sound tone typical for a fax message. Still upset and shocked by the news of the attack, I went to read the fax that just arrived.

My heart stopped for an instant.

That piece of paper caused an explosive reaction in me. All the explosions in the world would not have created a worse disaster. It was from Jorgos. He wrote that he could not go on with our story. He simply did not have the strength.

Full stop.

I waited for my friend and her funereal news to leave the shop and called him immediately. He could not get away with it like that. He would at least have to explain something more. Such a way to end a love story would be too bleak for anyone: after two years' worth of relationship I was entitled to a final phone call.

Reading the end of our history—and probably of my life as well—on a piece of paper was not acceptable.

Not for me.

The reason was always the same. A refrain heard and repeated millions of times throughout history. He could not fight against everything and everyone in order to defend our relationship. He was being criticized wherever he went, by whomever he met.

In any case, the decision was made, the die had been cast. He still felt very much for me, a whole lot, but he just could not face the idea of a future together. Everyone was telling him that he would regret it forever.

And how could I blame him? If the whole world whispers in your ear that you're wrong, in the end you end up believing it too, in spite of all that there had been between us: the nostalgic phone calls, the romantic surprises, the reassuring promises.

All wiped out with a sheet of paper—anonymous, cold, sterile.

I felt destroyed, annihilated.

How would I explain it to my parents?

What would I do with my life from that day onwards?

What was left for me after the end of my one and only love affair?

Nothing at all, that's what.

Yet, at the same time, I would not want to trap Jo in an unhappy future. In recent times, I'd had a glimpse of how sad life would have been next to a person who is absent, without the will to live, far more interested in friends than in his own better half. No, I did not want a life like that. Better for each of us to go separate ways, and what would be would be.

I did not want to live with someone whose wings had been clipped. Especially if the cause of that abomination was me. During that dramatic, endless phone call, I demanded just one thing: I made him promise that if he happened to change his mind, it had to be a final, definitive decision. If he chose me finally, it was to be forever.

That, at least, he owed me.

The news shocked my parents, who never imagined Jorgos to be capable of such behavior. For them he was still the wonderful lad who had welcomed me into his arms.

My mom did not accept the end of our story, and on her own initiative called Jorgos to hear the explanation directly from him. The news upset me because I would not accept anyone meddling in my life. I was quite angry and had a huge argument with her. She had to know that I was able to handle the situation, even without her intervention—especially without her intervention.

If nothing else, after that embarrassing phone call my mom was convinced that our relationship was over. From that day on she would devote her energies to support me rather than opposing me.

That was something.

A few days later, we started receiving anonymous phone calls. When my parents picked up the receiver, no one spoke on the other end of the line. Once I tried to answer first, but my skirt got stuck in the chair, so fate had it that my father did. And even then there was an utter silence on the other end. I interpreted the incident as a sign of destiny, like the good, hard-working fatalist I have always been.

Then, that night, the phone rang again.

This time I picked it up. It was Milena. Jorgos had just called her, asking for help. He wanted to know whether I wanted to speak to him or not. Quietly but firmly, I told Milena that if his intention was just to check out how I was, he could save himself the call. In fact, she told me that nothing had changed, but he was feeling bad about it and wanted to talk to me.

At that time I was still too angry to give Jorgos another chance. I knew we would end up in the usual argument, without anything changing in the end. I went back to my bedroom and started to cry. Bitter, helpless tears, just like those I had shed some time ago. Same taste, same intensity.

The next day I could not resist the temptation and called who by now had become my ex-boyfriend. Jorgos was grief-stricken and begged me to wait before making a final decision. As if it were up to me, of course. From that moment on his phone calls multiplied dramatically. His father would have had a new six-figure bill to pay, but the time on the phone line was well spent, and in July we decided to resume our relationship: we were still in love, and could not live without each other.

But a good part of the initial enthusiasm was gone.

In times of crisis, I had discovered sides of Jo's character I did not like at all: the nights out with friends, the drinking binges in company, the love for frivolous topics and the reluctance to face a serious conversation.

He was still the sweetest guy in the world, mind you, but with a hint of superficiality that sometimes worried me.

I had always considered myself more mature than my age. Inevitably, I had to grow up faster than others, to defend myself better from the outside world. OK, so I was too mature, too demanding, too deep. I could not expect the same from Jorgos. But sometimes I would have liked to talk about something more interesting than the usual topics: travels, football, travels, airplanes, travels.

I was already well aware that one day I would get tired of it all. One day I would demand a deeper, more concrete communication from him. But for now I had to be content, and thankful to still have an ongoing relationship. For everything else, I would have to wait for Jo to grow up.

Little by little—or, as they say in Greek, "*Sigà Sigà.*"

The turning point of our relationship was Jorgos's military draft.

In Greece, as in Italy, it was mandatory. Unlike in my country, however, the Greeks were forced to face fifteen months' draft because, by tradition, they felt constantly threatened by their neighboring traditional enemies, the Turks. Many islands were located on the border between the two nations, and were watched over by both parties for fear of an imminent invasion, which to my ears sounded absurd and ridiculous—surreal, more than anything else.

I actually had to change my mind soon: a few months after Jorgos had enlisted in the army, I overheard a small newscast in Italy, insignificant to the Italian people—except for me. A small Greek island, little more than a rock in the middle of the sea on the border between the two states, had been "invaded" during the night by the Turkish army, which had quickly claimed its possession, replete with a flag planted on the ground of that tiny piece of land in the Mediterranean. An international crisis ensued; winds of war started blowing but luckily calmed down soon.

From that moment on, I thought, I would rather not make fun of my Greek friends and their eternal rivalry with the Turks. The image of Jorgos at the front, with a gun in his hand, drained away any kind of sarcasm about it. It would serve me as a lesson.

Jo chose to pursue a career as a NCO, which meant staying nine months longer in the army. A nuisance for me, sure, but at least it would allow us to live together outside of the barracks, in an apartment of our own, a privilege granted only to graduates.

After an initial period of four months at a very severe cadet academy in Athens, Jorgos finally had the chance to choose where to spend the remaining nineteen months of military service: at the academy's school for officers he managed to reach the second place out of a total of eighty cadets.

I knew how hard it was for Jorgos to study. He had graduated in Vinci a few months after me, and it had been a real effort. Still, he liked the academy, despite his superiors' constant crazy yells and the fact that the cadets were not allowed to walk inside the barracks but only run. He told stories that made me cringe about life in the academy, but that period of very strict and dogmatic training did him well. He learned to behave in an austere and rigorous way, and I didn't object at all.

After the academy, Jorgos was again at a crossroads. He could choose either to be transferred to a barracks in Corfu, in order to help his father in his free time, or to any other destination, even thousands of miles away from his home, and be nineteen months alone with me, free from all the pressure that had ruined our relationship.

Once again, Jo chose me.

He asked to be sent to a beautiful island, far away from everything and everyone. We would spend the next months together, alone at last, in Rhodes.

Rhodes was the consolidation of our love story.

On that magical island, we spent the most intense and exciting months of our relationship.

We were united as never before.

We were sure of what we wanted out of life.

We would be together forever, and, if need be, we would move away from friends and family so as to preserve our love.

Maybe that was the solution, since our relationship was going better than ever away from Jo's family. We went out every night with other officers, their wives and girlfriends, and I felt completely involved in that small community. Whenever we could, we hung out on the beach or made trips around the island, in a sort of perpetual holiday. We were happy. Once again. *One-hundred-percent.*

Then, in early August, there came a phone call, the first of two that would end one of the happiest periods of my life.

Laura—Final Part

It was Mom.

She used to call me every week, but this time her call came too early. But I did not give much importance to the fact. Sometimes it happened. Mothers have their own needs, you know.

"Mom! Great to hear from you! I have so many things to tell you! I'm so happy, you know? Tonight Jo told me that we'll get officially engaged as soon as he finishes the draft. His parents agree with that. We'll arrange everything thoroughly, you'll see, and then we'll ... Mom?"

Silence.

"Mom, can you hear me?"

"Yes, I can hear you, Cri. That's wonderful news."

"Mom, what's wrong? Has something happened?"

Silence.

"Mommy, you're worrying me.... What's happened?"

Silence. A repressed sob.

"Mom ... Mom, please speak to me—"

"An accident—"

"Oh."

Silence.

"Mom, who? Rossella? Tiziana? Dad?"

"No—an accident in Spain...."

"What? In Spain? But who was in Spain??? One of my friends? Who???"

Silence.

"No. Oh, my God, no."

Very clear sobs.

"No ... no, no, no, no, no, no, no.... Laura? It's not her, right?"

Sobs.

"But it's not possible, Mom! She had to study! We invited them over, her and Gianni, we talked on the phone just last week, and she told me she had to study! They could not come because Laura had to do an exam in Spain—oh. Oh, God. Tell me how she is, please!"

"They are ... both seriously injured—There's not much hope— Cristina, don't come back. They are still there, in Spain. We don't know the details yet."

"No ... yes.... I don't know, no.... I don't know.... What am I going to do now? What do I do?"

I began to release a flood of tears. Torrents that would drain me over the following days. I called my sister, who told me the whole truth, which my mother did not have the courage to. Too much pain, too much, at one time. She had to dilute it in some way, at least a day or two, to prevent me from flying back home, or doing something stupid.

Rossella confessed that Laura and Gianni had died instantly, in a terrible head-on collision with another car, on a bend, in Palma de Mallorca.

Another island to mark my destiny, forever.

On that day, along with Laura and Gianni, a part of me died. As for Laura and Gianni, there was no hope left.

When you are touched by an event of this magnitude, Nancy, you can—no, you *must* declare time out.

I pulled out of everything. I lived through the following days and weeks in an atmosphere of utter unreality—extraneous and insensitive to any external stimulation.

Such a thing could not have happened for real—not to me, not now. When would I ever be ready to laugh, play, and joke once again? How long could a mourning so horrible last? Months, years, a lifetime? I lost the best friend I ever had, the most important, the most present.

Later on I learned that a few days before leaving for that damn vacation Laura had booked at the very last minute, she had showed up at my parents' house to pick up some ideas for the furniture. She had always liked the way we had furnished our home. She told my mom that she and Gianni would be married soon, and they had to start organizing things for the event. This news made my pain even more devastating, if possible.

I was destroyed, annihilated. The thing that troubled me was that I would never have the chance to see Laura grow up, step by step beside me, her life parallel to mine. I would not see her graduate and then get married, have children, and become a grandmother.

My Laura—my Lally as I used to call her—had been torn from life at just twenty-four.

All clear with a clean slate.

What sense did this all make?

And what kind of justice ruled the world?

Questions, questions, questions. Lots of questions, and no answers. Not one, ever, then or now. One certainty, though: the passage of Laura on this earth would not have been in vain. All the people she had touched with her presence had been enriched with an added value that no one and nothing could ever erase. Laura was a special being, and anyone who had met her even once in life would remember that precious jewel. A combination of beauty, gentleness and grace.

Laura would leave a huge void in my life.

I had loved her totally.

And I would miss her immensely.

I tried to return home for the funeral, but it was mid–August, and the flights from Rhodes were all packed with tourists who were not going to permit me to say good-bye to my best friend one last time. What's more, Jorgos did not want me to go back home: I was too upset and emotional. He tried to console me, but with no chance of succeeding.

I had lost the will to live. I was wondering all the time why such a bitter fate had claimed Laura.

She who had so much vitality, so much passion and so much energy.

She who had never asked herself what she was doing in the world.

She who had never blamed her mother for giving birth to her.

She who had finally found her way.

Why Laura and not me? Was it so hard to choose between the two of us? How could fate make such a huge mistake? How could this have happened? Yet I was still there, fighting like I had always had been.

Would there ever come a moment of peace?

I hoped so, because I was tired, exhausted, tried by life. Slowly, day by day, I would get back on my feet again, but the effort would be doubled and the result halved. Halved—that's how I felt. But I was alive, and apparently I still had to fight. Laura had wanted my happiness almost more than I did, and I could not disappoint her. I would show her, one day, that I had reached a milestone—my goal.

For me. For her. For our eternal friendship.

The finishing touch to the period spent in Rhodes, which started out idyllically and ended in such a tragic way, came on the first few days of the following year, after just five months of my personal drama. This time it was Jorgos who received a tragic phone call, and this one ended our stay on the island for good.

In Thessaloniki, after a desperate race to the hospital, his sister's 30-year-old husband, Angelos, had passed away.

Angelos, six-feet tall and over two hundred pounds of sympathy and smiles, the wonderful companion of jokes in a mixture of English and Greek which only we could understand, the new father of a little girl born just a few months earlier who was Angelos in miniature. Angelos, whose name summed up his entire being, had been struck down by an aneurysm.

We had to leave Rhodes and ask for an urgent transfer to Thessaloniki so as to help Natalie overcome such a tragic event. At just twenty-nine she found herself alone, with a child to raise, six hundred miles away from their parents and without a job to support her—a dramatic situation we would try to alleviate as best we could with our presence.

And so, once again, the great wheel of life had turned.

All aboard, ladies and gentlemen. Another day, another races.

Ceremonies

Jo's last months of military draft seemed never ending to me. A heavy-going period, exacerbated by an air of funereal gloom that permeated my sister-in-law's house and our lives.

There was a constant coming and going of friends and relatives who showed up to visit Natalie, trying to console her for a few hours during those endless winter days. I found myself in a situation of constant embarrassment, having tried so far to avoid any connection with Jo's family. Because of the old argument that had already cracked our relationship once, I had promised myself to stay away from any of his relatives until our relationship was finally stable: in fact, I had not returned to Corfu for nearly two years now. But that inauspicious event threw me right into the nerve center of the family. Into the heart of the clan.

The day of Angelos's funeral was a nightmare: a huge number of relatives, all dressed totally in black, seemed to be competing to shout their pain louder, louder and louder. Once again I was facing a foreign world, completely different from the one in which I grew up. I would have to absorb it and make it mine if I was going to live in this country for the rest of my life. But it was really hard.

In addition, during those terrible days I met dozens of people I had never seen before, dozens of faces that observed and examined me. They knew for sure who I was. They had heard about it, and now they could finally see with their own eyes the cause of such a sensation in their family. Fortunately Jorgos, who had not been able to stand by my side during those painful moments, assured me that everything would be fine in the end. I did not have to worry about anything.

It was selfish to think of ourselves in a horrible time like that, I knew it, but my future life depended on the reactions to those forced encounters with his friends and family. And I was lost in panic again, as the same fears came back cyclically, endlessly.

But this time I was wrong. Jorgos would keep his word. He would fight to the end. In December of that year that had started so painfully, we became officially engaged.

After the engagement, on Christmas Day 1995, our life together was stabilized. I spent on average two months in Italy and one in Greece or vice versa, depending on the period and the needs of the moment. The usual daily routine.

We loved each other, of course. But inside me the usual distressing doubts were multiplying. I was not convinced that it was Jorgos that I wanted. I had the feeling that I had to accept his behavior out of necessity, because I had no other alternative. I could not afford to wish for anyone else. I could never hope that the miracle might come to pass a second time. I would never find a new boyfriend—an ideal companion, well, that was totally out of the question.

I had to settle for the whole package, flaws included. These were the same ones that I had noticed in the past, in those times of deep crisis that had characterized our relationship. Jorgos was an eternal Peter Pan.

Affectionate, sweet, but with desires and dreams that demanded his attention all the time. He'd always want to be on the road. He constantly needed to move, explore, discover. And sometimes it was difficult to follow him. Sometimes I did not understand his need to get away from it all. His feelings seemed superficial, insubstantial.

But I went along with it. I had no choice.

And when I tried to get him on my side and engage in deeper conversations, focusing on concrete issues, he quickly got bored and moved on. I often locked myself in a room in the new house his parents had built for us and cried. I kept wondering if this was the life I wanted, if I could be content with what he offered me, without giving me the possibility of an alternative.

But the answer was always the same. In fact, it was a question: Who else would accept the syndrome and love me just for what was hidden inside me?

The years passed, along with my growing dissatisfaction. Jo and I had finally decided to get married, but I was tormented by a thousand uncertainties. During Easter 1998 I became completely alienated from everything and just wanted to go home. I almost fled from Greece, sickened by Jorgos's recent behavior. My fiancé disappointed me all the time. He made me suffer, wore me out.

He had added yet another hobby to his usual passions and threw himself body and soul into it. He had always loved the world of aviation, and since he had discovered the existence of a flight simulator, a computer program that reproduced in real time all the phases of an aircraft's flight from takeoff to landing, he spent hours and hours in front of the screen. Sometimes whole nights. For weeks he almost didn't consider me at all. I felt excluded from his life. I felt alone, misunderstood.

Once home, I told mom how much I suffered. I had decided to tell her everything, even though recently I had been trying to spare her any anxieties or worries.

Mom was not at all well.

She suffered from depression.

My mother had been a strong woman, energetic, unshakable for all of her life. Yet, for some time now, she had fallen into a strong state of exhaustion, which even resulted in a hospitalization. She made incomprehensible speeches that did not have any meaning. Fortunately, when the hysteric crisis broke out and Mom was plunged into the depths of her own personal black pit, I was away. Rossella decided not to tell me anything until I came back. From that moment on, everything changed.

My mother was unrecognizable. The medications had brought her consciousness back to normal levels, but from that day on she turned into a fragile, scared person. She worried about everything, in an obsessive and exaggerated way, and the smallest problem grew to gigantic proportions in her eyes. For this reason, we all decided to involve her as little as possible in our personal problems.

I never wanted to witness such a transformation. I had naively thought that my mother was a rock that nothing and no one could move, the reference point for the whole family. Now she had collapsed in no time, in an unexpected moment. Later on I found out that my mother's reactions to terrible events emerged only after some delay, when the adrenaline needed to address the present drama was beginning to wane and the emergency was solved. That was the moment of greatest weakness for her.

I had to start walking on my own two legs, because I would never be able to share with her my inner anguish and have her lead me on the journey of life. She could no longer stand, and I could not lean on the primary energy source of my life.

It was time to grow up, and do it fast.

Still, in the spring of 1998 I wanted to confide to my mother my innermost fears, trying to minimize the anxieties that had been haunting me for months. Especially because Jorgos and I were now very close to the fateful date: we were to marry that fall, on October 3.

It was time to organize the wedding: Jot down guest lists, choose the wedding presents and, most important, the dress. It was a huge thrill for mom to see me wear a white dress, the wedding dress, as beautiful as in a fairytale. We shed a few tears, despite everything. But at the same time my mind was clouded by bad feelings, weighed down by a sense of unhappiness.

After hearing my outburst, Mom told me that I would still be able to come home at any time, even after we got married. The wedding was only a formal act, I should not think of it as a life sentence.

Maybe she was right.

Maybe I should stop asking myself a thousand questions.

Maybe I should just go with the flow and be dragged to my fate, whatever it might be.

And so that May I travelled back to Corfu, filled with the best of intentions. I had not missed Jorgos at all in the month during which I had been at home—a unique and extraordinary event in all those years spent together. We had exchanged very few phone calls, and it did not bother me at all. No nostalgic thoughts, no complaints whatsoever.

I had built a shell of indifference that would protect me from his future behavior.

I was ready to do battle, armored and impregnable.

And then, in May 1998, after almost seven years of engagement and four months of marriage, Jorgos conquered my heart again.

For the last time.

My Big Fat Greek Wedding ... That Never Was

In those few weeks that we spent away from each other, Jo had undergone an amazing transformation. First, he had subjected himself to a strict diet, and returned to being the handsome and charming guy I remembered from the beginning of our relationship. But there was more. Day after day he helped me organize the myriad details of the wedding. He had collected the necessary papers at the consulate, chosen the type of paper, the font and colors to be used in the invitations, and taken me to visit the place where he thought the buffet and dancing should take place. And above all, he had found a perfect setting for the ceremony. It was a tiny church, all white with blue windows in typical Greek style, right in the middle of a tiny isle, accessible only through a narrow strip of land, a small footpath. From a distance, the church seemed unreal, magical. I was enchanted by it.

During the month of May, Jo was back to being the sweet, highly attentive person I had met seven years earlier. I was suddenly the center of his world again. No friends, no football, no planes or travels. I was the undisputed star of his life.

Jorgos was even able to suppress almost completely my eternal sense of insecurity towards the weaker sex: he made me feel so loved that I was able to dispel all the jealousy that I usually unloaded on him, with the result of making him even more in love, while I was even more radiant.

In a very significant way, I described May 1998 in my diary as the mirror image of the legendary, unforgettable July 1991: the absolute happiest periods of our relationship.

It seemed impossible to me that such a radical, sensational change had occurred in him. But Jorgos was really different. Maybe he had decided to stake everything on the marriage and take on his responsibilities, finally leaving aside the eternal child who lived in him. Maybe he realized it was the right time to grow up.

Maybe.

Or maybe not.

I did not want to go home after that beautiful, perfect visit. But it was necessary to return to Italy and bring the invitations to my friends and family, organize the wedding gift list, wedding favors—and solve at least a dozen other problems that I could not manage while in Corfu.

I visited a lot of friends to invite them to the ceremony in Greece. I told them how happy I was and convinced of my choice to move permanently to Corfu. And I was, I really was: everyone told me that my joy was transparent.

So much for my face's expressiveness. So much for the syndrome.

By the end of June I had collected eighty applications for the trip to Greece. We organized two buses that were to sail by boat from Brindisi to reach the celebrations in Corfu. An excellent result.

I never expected so large a participation. I had discovered how many people loved me and were eager to share our joy. Then, around mid–July, a week before my new departure for Corfu, the last trip that I would face before the wedding, I received a phone call.

Jorgos sounded distressed, different.

He asked a question that in a second blew away the pink cloud that had been floating for months over my head.

Wiped it out forever. With no hope of recovery.

I was suddenly plunged back into reality, against my will, with dreadful violence.

That question was almost like a slap.

"But, are we sure about what we're doing?"

The earth slipped from beneath my feet.

Just two minutes earlier, I had been the calmest person in the world—in the whole universe—and now Jo had fractured that so-hard-won certainty. How could he do such a thing to me?

I replied that yes, of course we were sure.

I was sure.

He was sure.

He WAS sure, wasn't he?

The day before he had been, so I did not understand what might have changed. Perhaps a moment of healthy, good old pre-marriage panic? Jo could not answer. But in the end he sensed how upset I was and yes, he admitted, that could definitely be the cause of his question. A legitimate fear, indeed. But I had to be quiet. After all, we would meet soon, and everything would go perfectly.

It took him a half-hour to convince me at least a little bit. Then, exhausted, he wished me a good night.

Ha, ha. Good one. Sure.

I spent a not very good but very sleepless night. I analyzed that question in my head in many different ways, through millions of different angles. My whole future depended on the understanding of that question.

I would not settle for a simple, banal explanation.

I would overwhelm Jo with questions, a thousand—a million—questions if necessary, to find an answer to that unique and terrible one.

I plunged back into chaos, into total panic. It would be tough to get out of it—given that it *was* possible for me at that point, be it tomorrow, the next day, or the one after that.

Or maybe never.

The next morning, at seven o'clock, I received a text message. It was the first time that such a thing had happened to me. It came on my brand new, bright yellow cell phone, bought a few days earlier to be up-to-date with the latest in technology. Jo had owned one for a couple of years, and it was time that I joined the modern world. And then, with all that traveling back and forth, it could be quite useful. If anything, it would serve to blunt my mother's by now pathological apprehension, as she would be able to reach me anytime, anywhere, at any second.

A rather convenient device. Not bad, after all, these mobile phones. Furthermore, they allowed you to communicate with short text messages. Nice—saving time, money and energy. Definitely a good invention.

The cute yellow object resting on the bedside table made a funny sound, different from the usual ring.

I looked at the clock. Seven sharp.

I was a wreck after that sleepless night. And I also had to figure out how to interpret the strange trilling.

Fumbling awkwardly on the keyboard, I was able to finally read my first historical SMS.

The sender was Jorgos, of course.

Cri, forgivve me. I did not want to hurt you. I love you so much and I want to marrry you. Forget the entire call. I can not wait to see you again. Everything will be all rigght. I love you. Your Jo.

The usual sweet, terrible, great, ungrammatical treasure of my life.

How could I not forgive him?

Yes, I thought. Everything will be fixed in the end. And then, there is so little time left. We are almost there. After seven years, the goal is near.

No doubt it will be just as Jo said.

In the end, everything will be *all rigght*.

A few days later I sat at the wheel on my Volkswagen Golf, which was overloaded with items and wedding gifts to be transported for my permanent move to the land of Greece. Despite all that I was about to leave behind in Italy—family, friends, memories—I was not afraid to face my new destiny, because there would be Jo at the center of everything. And to me that was enough.

On the evening of my arrival, we went out for dinner to a pancake house, a place I had always loved. I was eager to resume the "are-we-sure-about" topic as soon as possible, as I had to figure out whether Jorgos was ready for marriage or if he still had some doubts about it.

It did not take long to realize that the impasse of a few nights earlier, on the phone, had not yet been overcome.

We talked over dinner, between a salty and a sweet pancake.

He tried to explain.

I did not understand.

I was trying to extrapolate the heart of the matter, but we always came back to the same point: Jo thought that maybe we had been a bit hasty to make such an important decision. I tried to point out to him that our recklessness was the result of seven years of engagement. He agreed with me, but then fell into doubt.

I did not understand.

We went home and talked for hours, until sunrise. Jo explained to me that he had never known any other girl in his life, and he would never know if there might be "something better" for him. I patiently explained to him that, in the world, there would always exist something better. But that question, I added, might concern us both. I had doubts about it too, of course, but I thought that the love I felt for him would conquer all—without asking myself too many questions. He nodded, but he was not convinced.

I did not understand.

I tried to dissect the problem, analyze it under a microscope, as if Jorgos's crisis was a disease—or rather, a syndrome—that needed a cure. A quick, effective one, otherwise I would have risked losing the patient.

Was I losing him? Perhaps, I was.

And then we started all over again, with my process of detailed analysis, looking for convincing answers—that did not come but that he thought he had provided.

I did not understand.

At one point in the evening, a bat flew into the room and Jorgos ran away in horror. It was up to me to chase away the unwanted intruder. Ten minutes later, after a no-holds-barred fight by means of a broom, the bad bat, *i kakià nichterìda*, surrendered. Jo returned to the room and we burst out laughing to ease the tension. What a strange episode. A surreal scene in that extravagant night. He thought it was a bad omen.

I did not understand.

We fell asleep, exhausted, at five in the morning. I did not really sleep, though. I kept thinking, studying, extrapolating, and dissecting. What could disturb Jo so much? Was it really just premarital panic? And what life was waiting for me if we were to start it with all these distressing doubts? I certainly wouldn't want to force him, and trap him into a relationship he was not completely sure about. But what, what could I do to help him?

He was asleep.

I did not understand.

The next day Jorgos got up early to go to work and came back around noon.

I stayed in bed, experiencing for the first time in my life what it was like to fall into a real, concrete depressive crisis. My strength had left me. I was not going to leave that bed for any reason at all. The slightest movement cost me a superhuman effort. Better wait, and be still. And then, indifference to everything. A complete lack of interest, not to mention a visceral fatigue. Because of course, in the end, after all that effort, the result was always the same.

I did not understand.

We started talking again, about the same old topics, as though we had not tortured ourselves enough so far. Finally, after at least another hour of agony, Jorgos asked me a question.

"Cri, don't you think that there might be a specific reason for all this?"

I froze. I paused to think. I thought about it a good minute. Perhaps two. But no, no use.

I did not understand.

"Cri, don't you think there's a reason, the simplest of all, why I am like this?"

I looked him in the eye. I tried to read his thoughts. I had to think, calmly, coldly. I devoted myself to answer that question, I pledged seriously.

But I could not.

I was plunging into total darkness. In my head, nothing at all. No, not even then did it occur to me at all.

I did not understand. In spite of everything, I still did not understand.

"No, Jo, I don't know, I don't know what to think. You tell me."

And so he did.

I would never even come close to it, anyway. The truth was too far from my understanding. Light-years away from my small, naive, stupid enchanted world.

"Cri, I met another girl and fell in love with her."

Here it was. It had taken a while—a whole lot actually.

But finally I understood.

If someone had asked me, even just the day before, what would be my reaction to the idea of a betrayal, I would have answered—without hesitating or blinking an eyelid—that I would leave Jorgos immediately, not stopping to think it over. The first, huge lesson that I learned on that memorable day was that you can never really know yourself until you have to cope with the specific problem.

Assumptions are assumptions. I would do.... I would say.... All (excuse my French, Nancy) bullshit.

Another thing I thought I knew for sure was that if Jorgos did leave me, straight off, I would throw myself out of the nearest window or something like that. And I was totally convinced I would. Well, another huge pile of bullshit. Oops.

That day, that July 24, Saint Christina for believers all around the world, the absurd thought of suicide did not affect me in the least. Nor did I decide to leave Jorgos right then and there. No sir. The first crisp, crystal clear thought that crossed my mind was: we can fix this.

I, the pessimistic one by definition—the defeatist, the skeptical, negativity personified—generated a positive thought in that first moment of truth. Yes, I would fix everything, calm and cool. Don't panic.

From my eyes, which usually turned into a broken faucet for every trifle, not even the shadow of a tear gushed out during that crucial day. On that moment I felt like something had clicked in my brain. Something was off, or on, I would not be able to tell. I only knew that I had just undergone an internal change—deep, intimate, visceral.

I would never be the same person from that point on. I reacted with such dignity in such a dramatic situation that I really liked myself. A lot. I was 28 years old, and until then I had only ever felt self-contempt and self-pity: no character, no fortitude, no nothing.

But there had hardly been any problems to deal with. Real problems. I could not even know what was hidden inside me. Saint Christina, 24 July 1998, was the beginning of everything: a historic day.

Finally I had discovered that person who lived inside me. And I started to love her.

After the shocking sentence uttered by Jorgos, I took a few seconds to think it over.

I did not believe it was a joke, I could tell by his eyes that it was not. Then, I started asking questions, because at that point it became vital for me to get some answers.

I had to understand.

Lunch was completely forgotten. We stayed in our room all afternoon, to try and save what could be saved. Once I knew that there was a specific problem, I had to study it in depth, in all its facets.

I had to understand.

It was imperative that Jorgos explain to me how it had happened, where, when. I would examine the reason by myself, later on, if in the meantime he provided all the information.

I had to understand.

I had to know whether it was a recent incident or if it went back a few months. I had to know whether it had been by chance or a sought-after adventure. I had to know whether she was a tourist or a girl from Corfu. I had to know whether it was a one-night stand or a story that had a follow-up. I had to know whether it was all over or still in progress.

To know, to know, to know.

Every detail had become indispensable to me.

I had to understand.

But Jorgos was reticent and only answered my questions with mono-syllables. He claimed that it was no longer important, that the details did not matter. Well, they did matter for me, they sure did.

I would have to decide whether it was possible to overcome that painful stalemate or if Jorgos had come out of it as a different, transformed person.

I had to understand.

Then, at the end of that exhausting afternoon, by which time I had been able to collect some more precise information, while I was busy working out a solution to the impending disaster Jorgos delivered the final blow.

With a beautiful smile, eyes sparkling with excitement, he spoke.

"Well Cri, now give me a good slap as well, because everything I told you *is not true.*"

Well. That was the point when I crashed. I felt a kind of crumbling inside, so much so that I could almost hear the sound of debris piling up. But no tears. No, not even then.

I begged him, pleaded with him not to do such a thing to me and tell me the truth, immediately. I could not bear a lie so colossal and did not deserve such behavior. I would have preferred a thousand times to know everything at once, rather than live forever in doubt. Suspicion would kill me slowly, day by day. I pleaded, begged him to be honest. Jorgos was smiling, cheerful, relaxed. He swore over and over that he had made everything up just to put me to the test, and see what my reaction would be. I passed the exam with flying colors! What a beautiful thing, is it not?

I kept inviting him to consider what he was saying. I was very fragile at that moment, and he could break my heart with a whisper. Was he really certain of what he said?

Of course he was—he had even organized quite a complex plan, well thought-out for a long time. The imaginative recital had started with the phone call that chilled my blood just before I reached Corfu. The first act of that funny, oh-so-funny play.

Too bad I did not feel like laughing, not the least bit.

But Jo continued to swear. And swear. And the need to believe in his words, as unbelievable as they now were, was so strong. It was something that I needed to hold onto as if my life were at stake. And so, that night, I decided to give our relationship another chance.

I teleftèa, as the Greeks say. The last one.

Dawn in Paxos

The next day Jorgos hastily organized a trip to a small island south of Corfu. To celebrate, he said. To spend two days away from everything and everyone. Just for us.

Paxos was a beautiful, intimate island: it was just perfect. Still, I felt a little upset from the day before. Well, quite a lot in fact, but I tried not to think about anything and kept pushing away the bad thoughts whenever they crowded my mind—at a constant average, that is every five minutes.

I reproached myself silently: I was the usual pessimist, the usual self-hater, and the usual defeatist.

I was bad, bad, bad.

A boy who had proved himself so mature as to conceive such a spectacular set-up did not deserve that reaction. He did not deserve my obtuse distrust.

We spent all day at the beach, and I saw Jorgos sinking slowly into an invisible cloak of sadness, hour after hour. In the evening he had turned once again into a taciturn, pensive being.

"Jo, listen. I'm asking this again and then I promise you that we will not talk about it anymore, for a lifetime. I need to know if you've had an affair with another girl. At least this, you owe me. Then we'll talk about it all you want, but I need the truth."

"Yes Cri. There was another one. It's all true. Yesterday you reacted so well that I thought I loved you like never before. I thought I could fix everything. But I cannot. I am changed. Now I know that I can have any girl in life. I can no longer be content with you. It would not be right. But if you want us to go ahead anyway, I will. I can forget everything. The decision is yours."

"Decision. Yes, Jo, we need to make a decision, of course. We cannot pretend that nothing happened. At least I could not—ever. This story would be the elephant in the room. Sooner or later it would come out in any argument and it would be a disaster. And then—I will not lock you in a cage. You must have the chance to choose what you prefer and have other experiences. I think you'll end up hating me if I do not grant you a possibility. It's over, Jo. *Terma*. Enough."

We talked again all night, in the small apartment we had rented just outside the village, on the hills.

I was shattered, literally. In those last days I had hardly touched any food and I still remember the feeling of constant, insistent thirst that gripped my throat during those two days in Paxos. After that last conversation, I grabbed a bottle of water, and despite drinking from it every two minutes I could never quench that sense of dryness. I still remember it perfectly, a feeling I had never experienced in my life before.

It was like having a desert inside me.

At four in the morning, I found myself still awake, while Jo had peacefully fallen asleep a few hours earlier.

I got up and went to see the sunrise on the balcony of our small apartment with its sea view. In absolute peace, in front of that postcard-like picture, sitting on a chair with my eyes unfocused, I took the first crucial decisions.

I had to delete everything and start from scratch.

It might seem absurd, but I was not worried about myself. Or at least, what my life would be from that moment on was not my main concern. I had a much more serious problem: I did not know how to tell my mother about it.

She had called just two days earlier, on my arrival in Corfu, and did not suspect anything. I had carefully avoided telling her about the phone call I had received when I was in Italy, just before leaving. I could not risk her being worried unnecessarily. By now I had learned to hide most of my fears and anxieties from her.

My mother had become a frail creature, poised between normality and disease. Depression was a monster, attentive and quiet, crouched on the sidelines, waiting for a small misstep, ready to attack ruthlessly and cruelly at the first opportunity. I was sure that such dramatic news, just two months away from a wedding that had already been planned in every detail, would destroy her. Maybe not right away, but sooner or later, my mother would fall into a deep abyss, with little chance of recovery.

And then there was my father. He loved Jorgos and always regarded him as a son. He took his side constantly, in a spirit of camaraderie among men, even in indefensible situations. He would accuse me of engineering the disaster, I was sure about that. For better or worse, he would think that it was all my fault, with all that would then ensue—my mother's depression included. All because of me.

Well done, Cristina.

This and many other thoughts crossed my mind on that July morning on Paxos, Greece, an island in the Ionian Sea.

I was getting ready for a new life, new battles, trying to scrape up the little strength I had left.

Because from then on it would be needed, in large quantities.

And yet it was only the beginning.

Back to Square One

We went back to Corfu the next day, and I stayed with Jorgos one more week, to organize as best as I could my permanent return to Italy. As soon as we got back, my father-in-law took me aside by the hand and told me that he was ashamed of his son's wicked behavior. He was crying—I had seen him in that condition only at Angelos's funeral.

He told me that when the day came when I was a happy woman, I must call him and share my joy with him.

I promised him that I would. *Orkìstika*. I swore it.

Then I called my sister. I did not have the courage to speak with my mom, and I wanted some objective, thoughtful advice, so as to create the least damage possible to her fragile condition. I tried to reach Tiziana, the one with whom I spoke more openly about emotional issues. The one who always listened and reacted positively to all my confidences. As chance would have it, I did not find her. So I called Rossella, who, upon hearing the news, reacted with her typical seraphic calm and told me something that I would never forget, that would stay forever in my heart, just as, when a child, I welcomed her words of advice and her reproaches as indisputable judgments.

Rossella was a staple, a rock. She was the word. And she made me aware of a big, indisputable truth.

"Cristina, listen. If such a serious thing has happened to you, it means that a better future is waiting. Good will emerge from this episode, eventually. A person like you, with your problems, does not deserve to suffer. Someone or something saved you from an unhappy life. You just have to have patience and wait. At the beginning it will be hard, but you must know that you are in for a life a thousand times happier than the one you were about to live. Believe me."

And I believed her, completely. Rossella had always been a pragmatic person. She was my sister, and she would never lie to me—ever. That one certainty in my heart would form the basis of my rebirth. Now I could tackle any obstacle.

I would phone my mother, first thing.

I was finally ready.

Everything went just as I imagined. Mom tumbled from the clouds, having never suspected even the slightest whiff of crisis between us. For that matter, I hadn't—until a few days earlier. I explained to her that Jorgos had changed, and he would never be again as he had been. He had gained awareness, courage and determination, and could no longer live with someone *like me*, who had to offer only physical issues and endless problems with the entire family community.

It was sad, but that was that. And we had to accept it. I, for one, understood Jorgos. And I defended him, because in any case, in the past, he had tried. He had really believed in our love. But, in the end, he had to face facts. With me, he would never be completely, *one-hundred-percent* happy. Never.

I told my mother not to worry, as I would be back soon and we would have all the time we needed to talk calmly. My father decided that he would join me in Corfu and take me back to Italy. He would not allow me to come back all alone. He would help me load a second car, his own, with all my stuff to take home. His presence would be a great comfort. What's more, he wanted to talk with Jorgos one last time, eye to eye.

He, too, like me a few days before, wanted to understand.

The final week I spent in Corfu did me a lot of good.

At that point, it was not important anymore to keep his affair secret, and Jorgos told me about it in every detail. In that week I became his best friend: I listened to him, did not judge him, tried to be understanding. In any case, it would not have done any good if I had gotten angry. Now everything had changed, and we had as well.

I was amazed by my own coldness and lucidity—as if that hallucinating story did not concern me but a close friend of mine. Day after day, I discovered that I was able to withstand any news, any event. I had my life in my own hands, and I would not let anyone convince me otherwise. What is more, Dad defied all my predictions.

He came, made his speech to Jorgos—a speech steeped in bitterness and disappointment, as expected—and had the answers he was looking for. And he did not think even for a minute that I was somehow the guilty party in that situation. My father was on my side; he was with me.

In that one day spent together in Corfu, a small miracle happened. I realized I did not know Dad at all. Mom had always acted as a filter between me and him, and I never realized that behind so much motherly advice, often there was his voice speaking. Secluded, discreet but present. We had never really talked until then—never in a serious, thorough way. The countless times I called home and he answered, I used to kindly ask him how he was and then to pass me to Mom. Until then, I had never truly communicated with my father.

Then, in Corfu, I had a revelation, a very important one, and I had to thank Jorgos and his unexpected betrayal for that. My father was a *cool guy*.

That day we talked a lot, a whole lot. We made up for almost all the time lost in the past. And I discovered that he knew how to listen and—surprise, surprise—he could also provide answers. Wise, thoughtful, profound ones. Just like a best friend.

I told him everything, from beginning to end. It was the first time I shared that sad story with someone. It allowed me to lighten a small but important burden, the first fragment in a long series that I would gradually release in the following months. And every time I told a friend my story, I lost a particle of cosmic heaviness.

Yes, my father had been a revelation. The second in importance after the main one.

The main one was that I had finally found myself.

Good-byes were not particularly poignant. No tears, no regrets.

Jo asked me for one last time if I was quite sure of that choice, as if everything depended on me.

I was increasingly sure, indeed. We had both turned, each for different reasons, into two different people. Not strangers, no—rather acquaintances, old friends who discover that after years of living side by side they do not have that much to share any longer.

And that's how we would remain forever.

I did not hate him; I have never thought such a thing. I would always retain fond memories of him for all the battles he had fought to defend our relationship, and I would feel a sense of infinite gratitude for taking me away from a shapeless and meaningless life. No hard feelings, indeed. Jorgos had filled a huge void, a fundamental part of my life, and for this I would be eternally grateful to him.

Già pànta. Forever and ever.

The voyage home was a nightmare.

My father's car and mine were overloaded with personal belongings. I never thought I had transferred such a large part of my life to Greece, and still I had left many objects behind me: the most significant ones, which would have caused only unnecessary suffering. I had already embarked on the meticulous work of self-preservation, which from that moment on would characterize my every move, my every action. I had to prune, prune every twig that might annoy my fragile balance.

I had to save myself this time, before anyone else.

I had to love myself, and do it madly.

I had to put my emotional safety above any other purpose.

So, no photos, no videos, no tangible reminder in my suitcases. Objects imbued with memories had to stay away from me and my new existence. After all, it was a matter of life or death.

The ferry that took us back to Italy was packed full of people, so much so that one could barely move. Passengers bivouacked at every possible angle, making the air stifling, suffocating. It was the first time in many voyages that I happened to be in the middle of such a stressful, almost unbearable situation.

After twelve seemingly endless hours, compared to the eight expected, the ferry finally arrived in the port of Brindisi. There, we stopped to refuel the car before facing the almost four-hundred mile drive that would bring us home. As we left the station, a scooter came out of nowhere with two teens on board without helmets. I noticed them at the very last second and could not do anything to avoid them. The two fell tumbling to the ground, and with them my spirits also collapsed. I burst into a hysterical and uncontrollable fit of tears.

The lads were not hurt, however, just a few scratches. Dad got out of his car and promptly settled the whole issue in a few minutes. I stayed in the car, my head down on the steering wheel.

I was a raging river. A sea. An ocean. And I shed all the tears that I had not cried until then. I was ashamed to show myself so weak before my father, but I could not stop myself, I just couldn't. I was wondering if there would be an end, if I would die from dehydration, with all those tears spent.

That was the lowest point I have ever touched in my life. The darkest moment of my existence. The bottom of my personal barrel. Everything looked bad, disaster awaited at every corner. I could feel only negativity, in continuous waves, and I was beginning to think that there was no hope.

Everything was finished.

Game over.

To tèlos. The end.

Dad patiently allowed me a few minutes. He did not speak; there was nothing to say. He simply understood my pain and shared it, but he was powerless against that rising wave of anguish. Then, when I finally calmed down, he told me that from that moment on I had to follow his car step by step. Whenever he used the indicator and overtook a car, I would do the same. Whenever he changed lanes, I would change lanes too. Whenever he slowed down, the same he expected from me.

He suggested I just stay focused on the license plate of his car. Whenever I got distracted, I would have to bring my eyes back to it and read its numbers and letters, and if I were not able to distinguish them, that meant I was either too far or too close and had to bring my car back at the correct distance. The important thing was to keep my attention focused on the trip and not let the mind get lost in other thoughts. It was excellent advice, as I would not have been able to drive even a mile more had he not been driving ahead of me, leading the way like a luminous beacon.

I remember almost nothing else of that trip. I think I drove miles and miles just by mere inertia, simply following his advice. I had no strength, no energy, and could not think of anything. I just felt a huge void inside, like a black hole that sucked in every emotion. Overall, I was not fully conscious but merely an automaton—a machine inside a machine—with another one ahead of me, which I had to follow.

And I did.

Whenever it turned right, I turned right.

Whenever it turned left, I turned left.

And I kept staring at the license plate. Every two minutes I forced my eyes back to it, as if it were a matter of life and death, and it was the only thing left for me to do in life, my one and only goal. Never lose sight of those numbers and letters. Even today, they are burned on my brain.

AK 326 ST

We arrived home late in the evening. I was exhausted, but I had done it.

Mom did not say much. She imagined how tired I might be, and did not launch into the array of questions that I feared. In fact, she asked me to sleep with her that first night, taking the place of my father. It had not happened in at least twenty years or so.

I told her that it would not be necessary, but she really wanted it, perhaps more to comfort herself than me.

And so, that night we slept together.

I had imagined to go through another sleepless night, and instead, on that first night at home, I fell asleep almost immediately, hugging my mother. Physical and psychological exhaustion had done a good job in the end.

I regressed to the stage of a defenseless child, but it would be the last, final opportunity that I would allow myself.

Then I would start to live again.

THREE

Like a Butterfly

Going Down

The next morning, August 1, 1998, the first day of the month, the first day of my life without Jorgos, I made a decision—the first one. I would not let my mom see me sad, ever. I would turn the feeling knob to the notch marked "joyful and carefree." At least, on the surface.

However true or false it might have seemed, I was interested in the end result. I could not let my mother slowly slip into a depressive state from which she would never be able to recover. I put all of myself into it. When I came back home after work I always tried to have funny anecdotes to tell her. I often went out in the evening with friends, so as not to give the impression that I was locking myself in with my thoughts and problems. From a perennially taciturn daughter (Mom used to reproach me: you never tell me anything!) I had turned into a chatterbox, even logorrheic at times. And I always showed myself as being full of energy, even when I did not have much to spare.

Anything and everything not to have my parents worry.

And her. Most of all, her. The person that had loved me the most, the one I loved the most in the whole world.

Mother.

It was no use.

I watched helplessly as her mood declined day after day. She was fading like a candle under a bell jar. She lacked oxygen; she was being extinguished. And the worst thing was, we just couldn't do anything to help—not me, not my father, not my sisters, not her friends. She was no longer interested in any of us. She was isolated from us all, and it was an immense effort for her to perform any actions, even the most trivial.

Once a neatness freak, she was no longer concerned about the house or about caring for us, the other inhabitants of the house. In the end she had taken refuge in the only place that gave her comfort: the bed.

Never one to pass up a good gossip, now she almost did not talk to anyone. She did not even want us to visit her in the room. She who had always loved watching programs on TV, now lay for hours and hours in the dark, in front of a blank screen. She who had always had weight problems lost more than forty pounds in a few weeks. At night she did not sleep, as my increasingly worried father explained.

The situation was getting worse and worse, and we did not know how to help her. None of us had any experience of depression.

I tried several tactics, all equally useless. I tried to go along with her, just keeping her company, in silence. I tried to shake her, relying on her pride. I even tried to get mad at her, rebuking her and telling her that such a behavior was shameful. No avail. She was completely divorced from reality.

After about a month after my return to Italy I realized that I had lost her for good. The mother whom I knew no longer existed. That was the moment when I cut the umbilical cord that still bound me to her—a bond so strong that I thought it was unbreakable. In those days, when I needed my mother more than ever, she had abandoned me to myself. Or perhaps she had challenged me, and her inertia moved me somehow.

And I began to fly solo.

I had the strength; I could afford it.

Enough of childish excuses and useless whining. I was perfectly able to take care of myself. I had become an adult, and as such I had to act from now on. I was proving it to myself day after day. I did not complain about what had happened to me, did not cry, and did not have second thoughts, doubts, and perplexities. I had made a choice and I felt full of energy—and every time I told my story to a friend, it was like I was charging myself with more energy.

I liked to think that I was the master of my fate. This time I made my choice, and I did not accept any compromise. Enough of humiliations and submissiveness.

I was worth so much more, and no one would have me choose between myself and another, as from then on I would always choose myself. Because I had been good, having not collapsed. Because I was strong, having not fallen into depression. And I would have had reason to, as much as my mom. I would never find anyone who would want to share the rest of his life with me. I would be left alone again and for good.

Back to square one. But I did not care. Better alone than crushed by compromise.

My mom, the strongest woman I've ever known, had given up. I would never do that. I would never allow it. I walked a path opposite to hers. I had been weak, unable before to react; but finally I woke up from that soporific torpor and loaded myself with power, vigor, and vitality. It was as if my strong-willed mother's character had moved inside me, simultaneously abandoning her body.

Now I could "bite the next," as she had advised me one day, many years earlier.

Now I replied to the attacks of ignorant people and made them shut up.

Now I was not scared of anyone, not anymore.

Now I walked head-on, because finally I knew I could do it.

I liked this transformation, although I reproached myself that it came a bit too late. I did not even know whether my mother would be able to notice. That fortitude she so much wished to infuse in me was now mine, and yet she was not able to appreciate it. Not that or anything else.

Mother was absent, having taken a break from life.

Double Zero

Despite everything, I was not suffering—or at least not as much as I expected. Perhaps concern for my mother's depression choked every other feeling.

I had literally thrown myself headlong into work. I liked it, I always did, but now I loved it viscerally. I perceived it as an instrument of retaliation towards life. I would prove I was worth something, at least as a professional.

Rossella had managed the shop successfully, despite my many absences over the years, and besides the fact that she was also taking care of her wonderful children. When we opened for business Elena was just little more than two years and Samuele was only seven months old. Now that I was back I found they had grown up, and I realized that I almost did not know them. I had missed so many phases of their young existence. Birthdays, holidays, games, laughter.

I realized, as if waking up from a dream, that for seven years I had been completely absorbed by my story with Jorgos, and hadn't noticed what was happening around me. And I was ashamed. Very much so. How

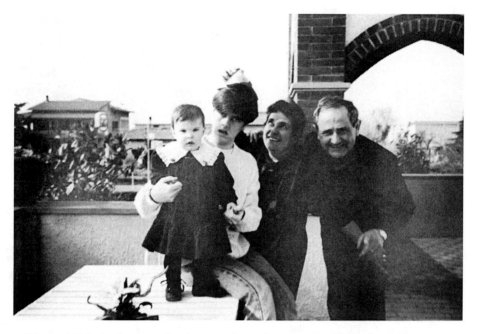

Winter 1990. A photograph taken on the patio of our home, with my parents and my niece, Elena, who was then just one year old.

could I have been so selfish? I thought only of my personal well-being, and neglected everything else. My parents, for example. How much had they suffered from my continual absences? How much did I worry about their feelings? The answer to the second question was cruel, but real: little, almost nothing at all.

Of course, from time to time in those seven years I had been back home for a few months. But was I really present during those occasions? No, I did not think so. Apart from the time when I had confided to my mother my hesitations about the wedding, it was like I never really shared anything with my family. I excluded them from my life. I realized this only now.

The first week of October came and went without any major event. On the third day of the month, a fleeting thought touched me. I focused my mind on it while watching the weather forecast in the news. It was raining in Greece. The sun would not kiss the day when we were supposed to have married.

A real shame.

The next morning I went back to work, as I had been doing now for two months, without any particular thought in my mind. I had to categorize hundreds of customer files on the new PC, and it would take months, if I did not hurry. I had to catch up. There was so much work to do.

A seven-year backlog.

A few days later, Rossella told me that she would not come in to work. She had to take Samuele to a medical check-up: it seemed he had not been feeling well lately. In the last week he had looked a bit pale, and the iron-based medicines he was taking did not have any effect on him. A blood test was needed.

A nuisance. Little Sami complained about losing a day of classes, as he and Elena loved to go to school. They attended the second and third grade, respectively, and were very good students. I could not help smiling when I heard about that: it reminded me of something.

Or someone.

On the morning of October 14, I walked upstairs for the umpteenth time to my parents' bedroom. My mother did not even turn to see who had come to greet her. She maintained her position in bed, lying with her back towards me. I sat on the empty part of the large double bed and asked how she felt.

"Good," she whispered.

Nothing else.

Hooray. Another beautiful day of absolute emptiness and cosmic nothingness.

Eventually we had decided to take her to a doctor. If it were necessary, we would literally lift her from the bed. Her reaction to that news a couple of days earlier was the only one worthy of note in one month or so. She said that she would never take any medicine and turned over onto the other side. It was the longest speech she had delivered in weeks.

It was time for us to act in her place. Whether she was willing or not, we would take her to see a good psychiatrist. Medications could do wonders in these cases. Depression was no longer considered a social disadvantage, something intangible and indefinable, as in the past decades. It had been thoroughly studied, and it was understood that it could be treated with excellent results. And we would fight it, indeed. We just had to find the right path. And a good doctor.

I said good-bye with a kiss on the head to the woman who had been a source of inspiration all my life and went to work.

As soon as I came into the shop, I got a phone call. It was Rossella.

"Hello Cri."

"Hi, Ro. Are you coming in a bit later today?"

"Yes, I will. I'm in Perugia."

"In Perugia? What are you doing in Perugia?"

"I'm with Samuele, you know—they had to repeat some tests on him, there was something wrong with them."

"The blood tests?"

"Yes. They called from the hospital yesterday and told me they had to be redone."

"But—why not do the tests here? Why go to Perugia?"

"They said it was just a precaution. However, they just brought the results and ... the markers' readings are all messy."

"But ... but ... what does it mean?"

Silence.

"Rossella ... what's happening?"

"Cri.... Samuele has leukemia."

Silence.

Void.

Immobility.

Fear.

Terror.

Apnea.

Tachycardia.

Panic.

Everything in that sequence.

Each of these sensations would deserve a separate paragraph, Nancy—no, a whole book.

The wheel had spun another round, and this time a double zero came out. Win or lose all. Impossible to predict an outcome. I never thought that there would be problems so huge, so insurmountable. It seemed that the ones I'd had to cope with were already enough, but they were merely debris compared to the mountain that now loomed in front of us.

My life, our lives, would never be the same again. Facing Samuele's disease would change all of us forever. And if we wanted to survive, we had to start changing. Now. Roll up our sleeves and start from simple things.

Unfortunately, there weren't any that took me back to the starting point. How to tell a story like that to a depressed grandmother, now in the acute phase of her own illness? How to tell a grandfather who had poured all his attentions on that grandson, and had just lost a "son"?

At that time—I don't know how—but I immediately learned an early lesson. Never ask a question that did not concern the immediate future.

Which wasn't the next day or even the next hour. The future that I had to worry about would be, from that moment on, confined to the next minute. If I fell into the error of asking myself what to expect the next day, that would be the end. I would never squeeze a damn drop of water out of any damn stone.

I had to face a minute at a time. One only. Or I would collapse. I would be beaten from the start.

And along with me, my whole family.

Double zero. All lose, the dealer wins.

The first two months following the "double zero" day were frightening. When Rossella called me, she was still waiting to know the outcome of the first of an endless series of sample tests from the spinal cord. From that test we came to know that Samuele's leukemia was of a fairly common form but lethal to a very high percentage of children.

Rossella, the rock, the imperturbable, had faced the news with an unshakable optimism: it could have been a rarer, incurable form of the disease, and yet it was not. That is to say, a first glass to be interpreted as half full. In the family, we could never maintain that situation without the half-full glasses Rossella gave us every day. She was able to see the silver lining in every cloud. I envied enormously that wonderful gift. A gift from heaven it was indeed, since her character was always ready to catch the best part of things and see the light even in the darkest hour.

Samuele, in the hospital, would have to be locked up in an aseptic room accessible only to her, for two whole months. He would miss school, but the teachers would visit him in the hospital, just for him. Rossella thought it was an improvement: in his bedroom, in the intensive care ward, Sami had a personal computer all to himself, in the years when his friends could only dream of owning one—another exciting aspect of his situation, according to my sister.

In those two months, Sami received initial care as part of a national protocol in which his parents had agreed to enroll him. It was an experimental treatment, and he was part of a group of children who would test its benefits. The doctors did not tell us much about it, though. They never let slip a word of encouragement, no false hopes.

My dad was always filled with questions, like all the rest of us. The difference was that he could never hold them back, even though he knew that no one would ever provide definitive answers. Rossella did not pressure the doctors, figuring out that even they did not know how the course of Samuele's disease would run.

Each child was a story in itself. There were percentages and numbers.

But we did not even want to know, because they were only sterile statistics, useless to revive our hopes.

Samuele responded well to his first treatment of cortisone, a massive dose that brought the white blood cells back down to an acceptable level. Rossella called us every day, several times if necessary. It was a way of pulling ourselves together. In that hectic period, someone was there every day to cheer him up. If I was feeling strong, maybe Tiziana was having a crisis. If my father was down, then Tiziana called him and they had a little talk. When I was about to give up, my father came to the rescue. And Rossella, who never looked sad, warmed all of our hearts by calling us from the hospital, her voice always sounding positive.

Those mutual calls, those long talks, kept us together as never before.

Under such events, a family either becomes a whole or it disintegrates. There is no middle ground.

We became a single, compact block.

With just one weak point: Mom.

She had been told about it, eventually. We had tried to hide most of the news from her, but even she had noticed Rossella's absence, despite being adrift in her own personal sea of constant numbness. She asked questions. She had been told half-truths. Then father took her to see a doctor. She was given medical treatment, which began almost concurrently with Samuele's.

A mocking destiny. Both were fighting against a monster.

Sami, a blood cancer. Mom, a tumor of the soul.

During those dramatic moments, each of us in the family had a task. My father would take care of Mom, who was in need of it even more than a child. Tiziana would think about the shop, or at least she would help me in the most difficult situations. I had been entrusted with Elena, who had found herself without her mother and brother all at once.

In no time I turned from absentee aunt to hyper-present pseudo mother. I took my niece to school and took her back home every day. She had moved to our house for convenience, and since my mom was still on the mend, I prepared lunch and dinner for her as if she were my own child. During that period we made up for all the time lost in the past years.

Elena was very attached to her mother, but she was strong and never complained. She clutched the receiver whenever Rossella called as if her every breath depended on that object. She had never spent a day away from her mother, and now she was facing whole weeks without being able to embrace her.

A heartbreaking situation. But it was what we had to deal with.

Over the course of those first two months, Rossella returned home only twice: to pick up some clothes and spend an entire day with Elena. On both occasions I replaced her at the hospital, which was a devastating emotional experience. Samuele lived his days alone in the aseptic room, which could be entered only after sterilizing the hands and face very carefully. As an extra precaution, one had to put on a dressing gown, overshoes and sterile gloves before entering—and, of course, a surgical mask. A simple cold could kill the boy.

Even though Rossella had explained it to me in detail, the preparations made me very nervous. I was scared of turning into a deadly threat to that fragile human being I loved so much. But Samuele was in high spirits, and when he saw me, he hugged me very tightly. I was afraid to touch him, even terrified, but in the end I relaxed and returned that heartbreaking embrace.

I had promised myself not to cry. I made it by the skin of my teeth. But then, in the car on the way back, I let the tears flow. Samuele did not perceive the gravity of his situation, and if he saw me sad, he would not understand. Rossella had done an excellent job with him. It brought back to me the memory of when I was a child, and she used to turn every object into a game to help me pass the long hours spent with our grandparents. With Samuele she employed the same system, and improved upon it. She made sure that he thought of his illness as a wonderful adventure: something special, singular, and unique. And Sami was acting like a happy child, without any resentment.

The only critical episodes were the bone marrow examinations, in which doctors used a needle so big that it would frighten anyone. But even on those painful occasions Rossella had invented a game to distract her child, and Sami had not complained since.

I believe I have never met a person more "motherly" than my sister. Well, perhaps yes. Maybe just one. My mom.

December came, and with it my birthday and the end of the saddest year of my life.

My sister and the baby returned home after the first two months of intensive care, in mid–December. They moved to my parents' house for practical reasons. Staying all together was the best way to assist one another, because there was a continuing need of it, for each and every one in turn.

Mom was responding well to the treatment and had started to recover once her beloved grandson had returned home. She was slowly coming back to life and had finally realized how much she needed to help herself.

Dad checked that she took all her pills, from first to last. It was vital that she followed the cure step by step; otherwise it would lose its effectiveness.

But the most important event of all was that Samuele was with us again.

Once back home, however, our kid had to return to the hospital twice a week, for various cycles of chemotherapy, that is, if there were not any other problems that arose during the rest of the week.

Just before Christmas, he had a slight fever—just over 100 degrees, but that was enough to create an emergency. Rossella rushed to Perugia for his hospitalization, and so both were torn from us during the Christmas holidays, leaving a feeling of emptiness and anguish behind them.

Fortunately, the situation got better in a few days, but the doctors demanded that the hospital stay be extended at least until after New Year's Day. Rossella told us that an amazing Santa Claus impersonator showed up in the ward, making all the kids happy and cheerful, and Samuele wouldn't have had the chance to meet him had he not been hospitalized. Yet another half-full glass of hope, courtesy of Rossella.

That was the first Christmas of my life that we did not celebrate together.

The first. But not the last.

Climbing Up Again

I said good-bye to 1998 at midnight on December 31 with a cathartic four-letter word, without any sense of guilt, Nancy. I thought I had every right to it. That year would remain in the annals of our family as one of the worst we ever faced.

But 1999 did not promise anything good. During the first months of the year, Samuele was very often sick due to chemotherapy. He was taking medication in doses so massive that he could not eat anything, felt a continuous nagging nausea and often threw up. Sometimes he bled from the nose at the most unexpected moments. When I found myself in those situations, something seemed to break inside me. I did not believe that there could be such debilitating emotions.

Still, it was essential to react. On those occasions I took Samuele to the bathroom and tried to divert his attention onto any topic that was going through my mind. Not that we needed it: Sami was always very calm, the quietest of all of us put together. He had been instructed by his mother how to act in such situations, and often it was he who taught us how to proceed in the least chaotic way possible. No panic. Only a great deal of awareness and courage, in a little man just seven years old. Seven precious years that I had been foolish enough to miss. An enormity. I swore to myself never to make such an error again. What Samuele was giving to me in that dramatic period could not be compared to anything: pure love, reciprocated moment by moment.

It had an immense sentimental value that did not make me wish for anything else. It made me feel complete.

Then Samuele's hair began to fallout. Rossella had prepared us for that moment. We were told in advance, well in advance, that it would happen. But the shock was still huge.

My nephew and I slept in the same room, and when in the morning I got up and went to greet him with a kiss, on his pillow I spotted a growing number of sacrificial victims. Many small toy soldiers fallen in battle, each a little more than two millimeters long. My sister had taken steps to make the event as painless as possible, giving Sami's hair a zero cut.

At the same time, his face was swelling beyond belief. He was taking increasingly powerful doses of cortisone as the weeks passed. Suddenly that face became like so many others, those that Sami showed us in photos taken at the hospital with his new friends. In sickness, all differences in age, sex and looks disappeared. All those children looked so incredibly alike they seemed like brothers, all sons of the same mutual suffering. Those months were difficult, tiring, and endless. But in the photos taken during that terrible time, an element always stood above everything else: Samuele's smile. Unshakable, serene, patient. And submissive, just like his disease that slowly, after months of treatment, was finally retreating.

All that remained of my daily energy was spent at work. At the shop there were many emergencies to be addressed. The problem was that I just could not stand most people anymore. My impatience with them started after the disconcerting news of Samuele's illness. Some customers came complaining about problems so mundane that they aroused murderous thoughts in me. Having to cope with those ridiculous situations dramatically increased my nausea towards the common man.

Most people did not realize how lucky they were to live in a "normal" world and have an ordinary existence.

Indeed, in the end I did not ask much. To me, it would be enough to catch up with a regular life. A trivial, insignificant one. Whatever, just as long as there were no more emergencies to be faced. I was hungry for normality. I did not expect to be happy. I just wanted to wake up every morning without a one-ton stone pressing on my heart. Just that.

Yet, despite everything, I knew I was immensely fortunate. I knew that such a period would eventually be a beacon on my path.

I had returned from Greece aware of being changed enough, but now I felt that I had turned into a whole new person. A better one. And it would never have happened if I hadn't had to go through a lot of pain. The shy little insecure girl with millions of complexes and uncertainties who lived inside me had taken a long vacation. Indeed, she had embarked on a one-way trip. This powerful, energetic, strong-willed, self-confident woman had replaced her. And this new entity would never allow anyone to crush or overwhelm her.

She felt good, she was at ease with her soul and finally also with her own body. A stupid physical defect was not of any importance in a world where you could die from a cold. A physical abnormality could not and should not change anyone's life, because it had an infinitely smaller importance compared to the real problems of humanity.

I had wasted too much time pitying myself, asking my parents, my sisters, myself why the syndrome had struck me. There were no "becauses." I had been chosen at random, in the lottery that was life. Just like Samuele.

And now I could put all the issues, all the problems, in their proper place. Different shelves, ordered by importance.

The syndrome was insignificant. Ground floor.

My mother's depression was higher in importance, but not as much as Sami's leukemia.

That was on the top shelf in the "priority" department.

How much time wasted in feeling sorry for myself! I was ashamed, almost. And how much people's attitude would change when it clashed with my newfound assuredness. Some were even intimidated. I would not let anyone look at me in a funny way. I reciprocated that look with equal insistence, and if it was not enough I asked them if there was any problem troubling them. I liked making them uncomfortable, embarrassing them. They deserved it. They could not afford to judge me. They did not understand what I had to deal with day after day. They could not imagine the energy that was needed. They just did not know me at all.

As an Indian proverb said, before you judge a man, walk a mile in his shoes. The new Cristina would never beg for other people's approval. If anything, it was the others who had to be special, greatly above average, to be accepted by me. I would be very severe in my judgments. And I would come up with them only after walking for many miles in their shoes.

Operator Forty-Four on the Line

This renewed security, this positive energy, was something that I could pass on to my friends, as if they were to need me and not vice versa. But there were also times when I lowered my guard and was immediately seized by doubts and anxieties: what would I do in my life now that I was alone again?

True, the moments when I could pause and think of myself were still too rare, but over time the usual problems would resurface, and I had no idea how I would react then. For the time being there were other priorities, I'd think calmly about the rest, in due course.

Then, in May of that year, something happened that would bring a little more turmoil in my life. A negative episode that eventually turned into a good story to tell. Yet another example that every cloud does have a silver lining.

One day at the shop, before returning home, I found out that my purse was missing. I tried to focus on events and understand how it could have happened. There had been so many customers that day and probably, in a moment of confusion, someone noticed the bag and stole it.

I felt bad about it. Very bad. It was the proverbial last straw that breaks the camel's back. Nonsense compared to all that was happening to me at that time, yet it unleashed a huge inner discomfort. For a whole night I cried silently in my bed next to Sami's while he was sleeping peacefully. The fact that someone had violated my shop—the only place where I felt calm and protected, the only place where I thought I had absolute control on things—had me completely destabilized.

The next day I regained control of myself and started to make some calls.

All my personal documents had been stolen. I had already blocked my credit cards and checks, but I still had to get a new copy of my driver's license and ID card, in addition to dozens of smaller tasks. Among other things, I dialed a special number to block a phone card that allowed calls on unlimited credit.

On the other side of the wire, after a long wait that almost made me give up, Maurizio, operator number forty-four, replied.

His voice was warm and reassuring as he patiently explained what I should do to block the card.

Probably I sounded distraught, and in the end I told him that my purse had been stolen inside my own shop.

The phone call went on longer than necessary. It was pleasant to talk to a kind stranger who had no need to listen to my misadventures but who seemed to do it with sympathy.

Then, in the afternoon I got a call at the shop. It was operator forty-four. He called to ask if I was feeling a bit better. I was surprised. Gratified. He had really cared.

From that moment on, for a whole year, Maurizio became a constant presence in my new life as a single woman. I spent whole hours on the phone with that gentle and discreet voice, either during the day or at night, according to his shifts. We used to talk about big things and small daily events, which we liked to share with a feeling of mutual harmony. I told him my story and he listened carefully, sharing my emotions. A beautiful friendship was born, unexpected and surprising.

A song by Italian singer Lucio Dalla would have described it better than me.

"*La sofferenza tocca il limite / e così cancella tutto / e rinasce un fiore sopra un fatto brutto.*"

(Suffering reaches the limit / and so it erases all / and a flower is born from a bad event.)

Living on My Own

Nineteen ninety-nine was running out.

Samuele continued his therapy, but by then he had started school again because now he had to go to the hospital only once a week. The most difficult period was over. He responded very well to treatment, but we could not yet claim victory. The doctors said that we would have to wait at least another four years before he was officially out of danger.

Sami was a lucky kid. Many of his friends did not make it, despite following to the letter the very same medical protocol. We would never know why some children responded to the treatment differently from others, but it was a fact. Only a matter of fate.

One of Samuele's little friends, for example, had had a complication a short time before. His catheter, a tube inserted into the chest to allow him to be cured without having to continually use the drip, got infected. My nephew also had a catheter implanted in his chest—all the children in the ward had one. It had to be kept with maximum hygiene because it was a direct access to the outside world, with all that could come from that.

For Sami's friend it was fatal.

Whenever Rossella brought home news like that, we ourselves felt the burden of mourning of those families as if it were our own, without having ever known those people. In sickness, all those kids had really become like brothers, and they shared dozens of moms, dozens of dads, dozens of virtual grandmothers and grandfathers.

Still, that powerful system of mutual communion and fellowship was not always enough to perform the miracle of life.

Not always.

Sometimes it failed.

For days, the pain was immense for everyone involved.

We spent the last day of the century and the millennium New Year in Piazza del Popolo in Rome. We had organized a small trip with Rossella, my brother-in-law and their children to get out of the house and leave an extremely dark period behind us.

It was a nice idea but not unique. Several hundred thousand others had it. The square was packed full of people saluting the new year, an oceanic crowd united for a cathartic, joyful rite. We went back home tired but happy to have had that experience, which was now locked in the box of memories forever.

A month later, I made the decision to move house. The pressing emergency at home was now over, and I felt a strong desire to pursue a new, independent life, one that belonged only to me. My uncle, dad's brother, owned an apartment that overlooked the piazza where my shop was located. A perfect location. A wonderful opportunity.

And so, at twenty-nine, I went to live on my own.

It was not easy to convince my parents, especially my mother.

For some time now she had resumed in full her vital functions and social needs. She did not understand why I needed to get away from them—or simply she did not want to lose me a second time. Actually the distance between our house and the new apartment was a little less than a mile. But it was not the physical distance that worried her. She was beginning to realize that I had cut the invisible cord that had joined us for so many years, and she could not accept that her daughter had grown up.

There was a heated argument about it, which I still regret and am ashamed of to this day. It was one of the few times when I lost control with my parents. Angry words flew and nasty things said that I had never imagined were inside me. I spat out the poison and hurt them both. Probably it was an outlet for the stress accumulated over months and months of sleeplessness. In any case, they did not deserve such treatment, and the next day I apologized.

But it was too late for everyone—for me, as I would regret it for years, for them, as they realized they had lost me forever.

It's an episode that still grips my heart in an overwhelming vise. One of those things that I wish I could erase with a double stroke of the pen, even though I know that will never be possible. It generated a burden of guilt that I dragged behind me for a long, long time.

Living alone, taking care of myself, was definitely gratifying.

Finally a little bit of healthy selfishness. Just what I needed after my hard-won independence from the family.

It was a kind of rehearsal before the opening night. I wanted to understand whether that sense of liberation from the deeper bonds of affection resided only in my head or if it existed in the reality of everyday life.

Loneliness, which had frightened me so much in the past, was no longer a black monster to fight. On the contrary, it had become an accomplice, a life partner.

It took me just a few weeks to realize that I could take care of myself very well. It had been a year and a half since my return from Greece, and during that time there had been small moments of emotional crisis. But they were often swept away by the most urgent needs, which did not allow distractions of any kind. And it was good. Little time to think, very little time to suffer.

I had a few sporadic contacts with Jorgos that I thought about only marginally. That painful chapter was over and done with, and it would have been foolish to torture myself unnecessarily. It was always he who got in touch—because of several small practical issues still to be resolved. Those phone calls were useful to remind me that it would not have been a happy life, the one that I would have had in Greece.

Then, one day, a call came.

Jorgos informed me that he was going to make a trip to Tuscany to meet an old mutual friend, an enthusiast of ultralight aircraft. Jo was about to get a private pilot's license and would come over to discuss some technical matters with his Italian friend.

He asked if we could meet.

I thought about it all the next day, and I finally decided that it would be a good way to test my feelings.

Jo picked me up on his car and we went to a pub for a chat. We exchanged news about mutual friends, a long blah blah with no meaning whatsoever. Then he took me back home to my new apartment. I allowed him to come up and we settled into the living room, on the couch, looking at old photos.

And—There came a point when *we could*—

I remember formulating a clear limpid thought a moment before he tried to kiss me. If I allowed him to, I would contaminate my living room, the apartment, my new personal retreat, forever. From that moment on I would have to live in a place that would constantly remind me about that one mistake. And I could not let that happen.

I remember this. I remember myself escaping that dangerous kiss. The next day, in an excited phone call, Jorgos told me a different story. It was he who had escaped the kiss.

Rightly so. Each of us would hold onto our own truth. The most convenient way not to suffer.

Immediately after Jorgos left my apartment, at two in the morning, I picked up the phone. I tried to call my confidant, my new best friend. I looked for Maurizio, operator forty-four, with very little hope of success, because it was highly unlikely that he would be on a work shift on that very night. But I found him on the other end of the line, in his place, in my moment of greatest need. He was there, and he would listen and console me, as always.

Maurizio calmed me down. He assured me that I had done the right thing. It was an immense pleasure to share the same thoughts, the same feelings with him. Those daily phone calls allowed me to charge myself up for the whole day, waiting for the next call. I was in love with a voice, and I was fine with that. He could keep me company forever, if I wanted it.

But early that year, in my small rented apartment, I bought myself a personal computer.

And nothing was ever the same again.

I have to make an important confession to you, Nancy.

The Internet has flipped my existence. Upside down. Literally. A revolution as radical as it was unexpected.

From one day to the next, in February 2000 the World Wide Web, the window on the world, opened in my bedroom on the first floor of the apartment in Piazza Sandro Pertini, Civic number 17, in a small Tuscan village which very few people knew or had heard of, even in my own region. An ocean of possibilities unexplored, unimaginable and still inconceivable for my vivid imagination. A whole universe to discover.

The technician who installed the computer quickly explained to me what a search engine was.

"Excuse me, what?"

"Search engine. You enter a word and the system will browse for related topics and links."

"Excuse me, what?"

"Links, you know, those query strings that allow you to open new windows and surf on sites."

"Excuse me, what?"

And so on, for at least an hour. The most absurd conversation I had ever had. I felt incredibly ignorant, and I probably looked it. Never heard of that stuff before, just a few hints here and there. But I liked it. I was sure I would learn soon. I did not know that the Internet would be the turning point of my life. The decisive one. The last spin of the great wheel of fortune.

It would take a while. I would still fight and suffer. I would try and I would make mistakes. I would fall and I would rise again. But it would be worth it. A necessary path to happiness.

Thanks to the Web, one day a new presence entered my life. The most precious, exclusive, priceless gift ever.

My husband.

IKLY

One evening in March, about a month after buying the precious PC, I was intrigued by a small box on the side of the screen, in which a simple word, just four letters long, stood out.

Chat.

I had vaguely heard of it but had no idea what a "chat room" actually was. I clicked on it with the mouse, and a new icon opened, inviting me to choose a nickname.

Uhm. OK. Don't panic.

I would definitely not use my real name. It was dangerous. One can never know what might happen in such strange, unfamiliar places. And then, there was such wide choice of possible names. I would use one that I hated, so that if someone had to get into trouble, it would be someone that deserved it.

I chose the name Claudia, which by a very curious coincidence was also the name of the girl who had upset my life, two years before, by having a short-lived affair with my ex-boyfriend. Talk about chance, even if sub-conscious.

After a few seconds, another small window appeared out of nowhere.

"Hi."

Uh? Hi? Hi to whom? Is it to me?

"Hello." *Let's see what happens.*

"Where R U from?"

Huh ??? What? Ah, OK, I got it.

"Tuscany, and you?" *Better to keep it vague.*

"I'm from Puglia :-)"

OK, so it really exists. Someone is writing me from Puglia. But what are those two points and a half-round bracket?

"Cool! Excuse me, it's my first time here."

"Noooo, don't believe it! :-D"

"Um, sorry to disappoint you, but it is. Excuse me, but what are all these dots you use?"

"Lol. That's smileys ! Smiling little faces, you know."

Lol ?????? Gee, no I'll never make it. I'm looking like a nerd.

"Ahhhh, OK. But ... lol? What does that mean?"

":-D :-D :-D Laughing out loud! You crack me up! You really mean you don't know about any of that?"

"No, I swear, but I learn fast!"

Meanwhile, a second window opened.

"Hello, Claudia."

Who ???? Ah, OK, OK, OK, that's me, of course. And now what am I going to do with Mr. Lol ???

"Hello. Where R U from?" (*Here's the fast learner!*)

"Rome, and you?"

"Hey, Miss first time, R U there?"

Oooooops, help! What should I do ???

"I did not understand the question, sorry."

"I said are you still there—looks like you were gone!"

"I am, I am, but a new window popped up and there's a guy from Rome—"

"Claudia? Did you pass out?"

"No, no, I'm here. Could you please wait just a minute? I have a little problem to solve—"

"OK. Hurry, though."

Finally, a third, a fourth window. Within a few seconds I was in panic. A hilarious panic. I was having so much fun! Amazing stuff! Who would have thought?

At the end of that very strange evening I had obtained some important information:

(1) Mr. Lol's real name was Leo;

(2) He was chatting from a disco where he went to learn some Latin-American dance steps;

(3) He was of an unspecified age between twenty and thirty years old;

(4) He liked me a whole lot.

Et voila. A first virtual friend had been conquered by my explosive personality. And the same effect had also been observed in Mr. Hello-from-Rome as well as countless other Hello-friends that very evening.

They all filled me with compliments: I was very nice, funny, interesting. It was gratifying, but it was also dangerous. You could even end up believing all of it. And in time I would learn that compliments must be taken, weighed, calibrated, and then reweighed before finally being stored. And not without first having them roughly trimmed a little while round the edges, just to get them right.

But that night was my first time. I had wandered into it innocently, as with all first times. And it made me euphoric. I had discovered a new world. From a small room in my apartment I could reach anyone, anywhere, at any time of day or night. I could find new virtual friends endlessly. I would never be alone. Meanwhile, I had an appointment for the next evening with Leo, the aspiring Latin-American dancer. Same time, same chat room. Something to look forward to. Someone to talk to. Not bad for an object that had cost a few hundred thousand lire.

My first computer. And to think that it had seemed expensive!

In bed, that evening in early March in the year two thousand, I thought it was the best buy of the century. Indeed, of the millennium.

Just priceless.

The next day, Leo was punctual. Same time, same chat room.

He showed me two or three other new smileys that left me delighted. During our telematic conversation, other users intervened, and almost all introduced themselves with the usual "Hi" in a very original way.

I began to take the luxury of not answering every single one of them. After all, I could not allow them to share my precious virtual company after just a simple greeting: they would have to invent something better to win over my attention. Within just twenty-four hours I had become demanding, and I happily wallowed in my pond of virtual pride.

Leo was very cute and kept asking me a lot of questions. I immediately decided to make one thing clear. I wanted him to know that he had not come across Claudia Schiffer, as the nickname I was hiding behind might imply. I confessed almost immediately that Claudia was not my real name: that lie was easy to unmask. But it took me two more evenings' worth of chat to describe to him my physical condition.

That truth was a bit harder to share with a stranger. But I felt the need to be honest. It was a desire that haunted me, as if to hide my condition could have devastating effects. I could have pretended to be beautiful, hidden behind a screen, invisible to the eyes of Leo and the whole world. But I could not accept the idea of creating ephemeral illusions in my new friend. He had to know the truth, and then he would decide whether he was still interested in talking to me, despite everything.

Amongst other things, the syndrome was not easy to explain, not at all.

It was a *rarity*.

Very complicated to describe in a chat.

But I tried, and Leo declared that it would be of no importance to the progress of our new friendship. Moreover, he also had something to confess: he was not twenty-seven years old as he had previously stated, but twenty-two. He had not told me earlier because he was afraid that I might think he was a child, and he did not want to lose me over such a trifle.

Lose?

Oh, well, we could discuss that later, there was no hurry.

Indeed, he had proven to be mature. And anyway, a little lie would hurt no one, if it was for a good cause.

In fact—he agreed—"And besides, blah and blah and blah and blah."

"Certainly"—I replied—"But you know that, blah and blah and blah and blah?"

"Oww, come on! How cool. Yet blah and blah and blah and blah. And you know what? IKLY."

"IKLY?"

"I kinda like you, Cri."

Oh, here it was.

"How about you?"

"Me? Me what?"

"Do you like me just a little bit?"

"I guess so, Leo. IKLY too."

The days flew by—finally. A moment of respite after months and months of suffocating pressure. Each evening I came home from work and found e-mails waiting for me that would light up my day. Leo's were full of phrases written in bizarre fonts and bright colors. A feast for the eyes and the heart.

And then there were others. Friends I had met in the same way the following nights. And all, all of them claimed that the syndrome was definitely not a problem for them. They were a thousand times more fascinated by the way I wrote, by my feelings, by my character. None for the moment demanded that connected to such a beautiful soul there would also be a pleasant-looking body. Virtually speaking.

It was the first time that I was able to express what I had inside before showing what I offered from an aesthetic point of view. A chance of extraordinary importance.

A similar thing had happened on the phone with Maurizio, operator forty-four. On my computer, however, the opportunities that were granted to me were even more solid. I had all the time in the world to capture the sympathy of my new friends. I could attract dozens of people with my ability to communicate. Furthermore, I had a story to tell, dramatic enough to deeply impress the more sensitive souls. And all this without any need to show myself physically. A limit that had always ruined everything in the past.

For the first time, after thirty years lived in the shadow of the syndrome, I was finally able to escape it. And now I was out in the open, caressed by a warm and bright light.

Karim

Karim entered my life in small steps.

He was different from the others. The first night, during our very first chat together, he seemed a bit shy. Extremely reserved, introverted. And despite the little experience I had, those traits seemed like an uncommon thing on the Web.

Throughout the evening Karim answered in monosyllables during our virtual conversation. And yet, every time I got tired of his reticence and threatened to leave, he clung desperately to the keyboard and typed long, long sentences, trying to convince me to stay. A strange type—who in the end gave me his home number, if I ever felt like calling him.

It was a step that I still had not undertaken with any of my new virtual friends—not even with Leo. With him we limited it to exchanging our mobile phone numbers, and every now and then from his came nice short rings that I could not interpret at first. Then finally Leo explained that it was a way to communicate that he was thinking about me at that precise moment. Another novelty: I would never have reached that explanation by reasoning. Until that day I had used the mobile only for practical purposes, in cases of emergency. Now I had just discovered a fun use of it. How many things I was learning!

Still, there was a tacit agreement between us: no voice contact until I was ready to take that next step.

Leo was good with that.

And we were all perfectly happy that way.

Karim surprised me for the umpteenth time that evening. He did not seem interested in knowing me, and yet he left his telephone number. I was blown away. He took me by surprise, and he would do that again hundreds of times in the future. He was like that: an inscrutable mystery. I think it was this fact that attracted me. He had piqued my curiosity. He was like a closed book, and I wanted to be able to read him. It felt like a challenge. I had to conquer him. Serious business. After all, my infamous reputation as a "spellbinder" was at stake.

The next morning, a day off from work, I took courage and dialed the number. A beautiful male voice, deep and friendly, answered—but it did not belong to Karim. It was his younger brother, who informed me that I had to call an hour later. I waited two, just in case, before dialing that number again. But the phone rang and rang, even on the second attempt. It seemed I would not get to speak to Karim. I was about to hang up, determined to give up the meaningless treasure hunt.

The whole story would finally end on that very moment, since I had not left my telephone number, nor was I going to leave it now.

At the last moment, however, Karim picked up the phone.

"Hello."

"Ah, hello, it's Cristina, the girl from the chat room."

"Yes, hi."

"Hi again. Sorry to bother you, perhaps you're busy."

"No."

"Ah, OK. So ... how are things going?"

"Good."

"Good, perfect. Ehm ... were you going out?"

"No."

"OK, great, so if you feel like it we can talk a little."

"OK."

"Cool—But, are you sure I'm not disturbing you?"

"No."

"Well, if you keep answering in monosyllables, it is not going to be much of a talk."

"You see, I'm not good at talking."

"Damn, seven words in a row, one after the other, that's great!"

He laughed at my joke. Better than nothing. At least he was not the curmudgeon type. What an effort, though!

During that first, brief phone call, I made myself a pretty good picture of him. I did not think I would ever cross that guy's path again. Too shy— or detached. Or maybe just rude, who knows.

In any case that did not concern me. I had at least six or seven alternative contacts who had proven extremely loquacious and were quite willing to interact with me. I would definitely not miss that oh-so mysterious guy.

I just would not think about him anymore, quite simply.

That very evening, while I was virtually entertaining my friend Leo on our umpteenth chat, a new dialog box opened up. Instead of the usual "Hello" a very elaborate text appeared.

Karim started with a sentence that was more like a letter of apology than a simple chat message. He wanted to tell me, without my having any chance to fight back or stop him, that he had not behaved very well during our phone call and now he was asking for a second chance.

That was the moment when, even if unwittingly, I assigned a direction to the course of the ensuing months.

Answering to that message would drastically change my future. I started a chain reaction that would upset my existence once again. A butterfly effect that would hit me deep.

Because, after thinking about it a couple of minutes, I finally decided to give Karim a second chance.

In the days that followed, there was an intense exchange of messages via mobile phone and a complicated crescendo of phone calls, increasingly rich with confessions and confidences.

Karim was finally opening up, leaving the shell of distrust that he had created around himself. He kept amazing me: it was the first time that I was unable to decode a person's behavior. He kept me off guard all the time.

I could not read between the lines of his abnormal, cryptic communication. He fascinated me, but at the same time I was scared of him. Having to deal with a personality so ambiguous intrigued me but also caused me deep unease.

Meanwhile, the ice sheet that surrounded him was slowly melting. He began to flatter me with compliments, something I was accustomed to with my other virtual friends; but in his case they seemed sincere because they were hard-won.

The biggest mistake I made in those months of endless phone calls and messages was to stall for too long. I had left too much time without giving myself a chance to find out what would be the reaction of both of us to a real-life date. I should have met him earlier, but the same old fear of not being accepted because of my physical condition had grown inside me all over again.

I explained to him right away that I was not an ordinary-looking person. I also mentioned the name of the syndrome, and he searched about it on the Internet to find out what it was. He did not seem impressed at all.

He asked a few questions to which I responded without embarrassment, well aware that he had every right to run away from such a situation.

Yet he did not escape. On the contrary he urged me to look it up on the Internet to see if there was any kind of solution to my case. After all, a number of years had passed since the last surgery I had undergone, and none of us in the family had bothered to inquire about new developments in science.

And so it was that one day in the summer of 2000, while surfing the Web, I discovered the Italian Moebius Syndrome Association. It was Karim who gave me the right input. The only gift that I can say I'm grateful to him for. Everything else, however, ended up an utter disaster.

Feels Like Rain

The days overlapped, all similar in their extravagance.

Karim clung to me in an obsessive, almost morbid way. He gradually showed an increasingly intrusive and destructive jealousy. We had not even met once, and he already demanded that I not go out with friends. He thought it might be dangerous, and he was afraid of losing me.

I was dazed by such behavior, unable to deny him the respect he demanded so vehemently. But I realized that I was living an unusual, abnormal relationship, and a face-to-face confrontation was required as soon as possible.

We decided to meet in the place where he had moved to work: Germany, near Lake Constance. I would drive over there, so that I would have the means to come back at any time if I had to. For all I knew, I might also make a direct about-face as soon as I understood his reaction to our first meeting—his reaction to the syndrome.

I had mixed feelings about the encounter.

I liked the idea of being able to win over such an intense personality, I was gratified by his attentions, but at the same time I was scared of the energy he put into a relationship that was still only theoretical, virtual. Such an excessive involvement did not seem normal—especially since he hadn't seen me, not even once.

And so, about three months after our first contact on the Internet, I made up my mind. I was going to meet my destiny.

A blind date.

That definition turned out to be literal, as I was sending myself into a tunnel.

My parents had been told only some parts of the story. I did not think it was necessary to go into the details, as they would never understand. Moreover, I could barely understand it myself sometimes. It was a mistake, I felt it was, but I had taken a direction and I would follow it to the very end.

My mom was very worried when she realized how Karim and I had "met." She did not know such things even happened. I tried to calm her, but it was virtually impossible. In any case, I had become an adult, I had my experiences and my mother would have to accept her daughter's new identity. I had grown enough to be able to act autonomously, without taking into account either my parents' opinion or that of my friends—or anyone else, for that matter. I was going through the "my-life-is-mine-and-I-am-doing-whatever-I-want-with-it" stage.

I was wrong, but I did not understand that then.

I was full of pride for having overcome so many difficult moments. Full of arrogance and *hubris*—feelings that made me blind and obtuse. And selfish too, because I believed myself to be in credit with life. I had given everything to others and now I wanted to get something in return.

I was lacking self-criticism. I was losing my grip. All this was the result of that relationship that was dragging me away, toward a maelstrom.

I was sinking into a quicksand, one I still did not know the texture of.

The trip to Germany was horrible.

It rained from start to finish, and for long stretches it looked like a flood. I drove stubbornly, eyes forward, staring at my goal. I would not be discouraged by a few drops of water.

We were to meet at the train station in a small town that he directed me to by telephone. Karim was on time. As soon as I got out of the car, I saw him move towards me with a red rose in his hand. He was smiling as he approached.

He had two spectacularly beautiful eyes, emerald green.

He gave me a kiss on the cheek and looked me straight in the face. To me, it seemed like forced behavior, as if he had already planned it in detail. In one of our countless phone calls, I confessed to him that I could not stand the people who did not look me in the eye when talking to me. Now he was pointing those wonderful green eyes right at mine.

But there was something wrong.

We entered a bar to get something to drink, and the tension slowly eased. Now that he finally understood what I had been talking about again and again for days and weeks, he was calmer. The syndrome did not worry him much: I saw that from his eyes. But he was still scared and confused, and this too I felt.

There was something wrong.

We talked about the journey, how difficult it had been to drive in the torrential rain, almost as if the sky had decided to offload all the water that was at its disposal in a few hours. But I had been more stubborn than the sky, and in the end I won. I had arrived—I wanted to, I had to.

When we got up to leave the bar, I stopped to think rationally about the whole situation: this was not a spontaneous, natural meeting. I continued to have the same strong feeling, even when we got back to the car to pick up the suitcases and take them to his apartment.

There was something wrong.

Slowly, with small baby steps, the embarrassment that had dominated our first meeting was replaced by increasingly blatant and more spontaneous displays of affection.

In those five days spent together, Karim was an endless source of pampering and attention. After the difficult initial approach, the holiday was proceeding at full speed. We played the part of tourists in love, strolling around hand in hand in the towns around the lake..I felt so good that I had completely forgotten to call home and tell them that everything was going smoothly. Two days had passed since my arrival, and I purposely turned the phone off all the time, so as not to be disturbed. When I finally called home, my mother picked up the phone, and I thought she was going to cry with relief. And she never cried.

I quickly realized how huge a mistake I had made not to let them get in touch with me. I apologized in a thousand ways, but it was too late—another of those events that were simply irreparable. Lately I just did not seem to do the right thing with my parents—ever. And they did not deserve to be treated that way. I had been reckless to behave as I did, there was nothing else to add.

Mom eventually calmed down, but she would remember the episode, and from that moment on she would associate it with a negative feeling—to a negative person.

Karim did not have a good effect on her daughter.

When the time came to say good-bye, there were no particularly romantic scenes to take note of. The end of the holiday was acted out in the same way as it had begun: with embarrassment and insecurity.

I departed with the feeling that I had not left a special imprint on Karim's heart, but as always, he proved me wrong almost immediately. He called me on the cell phone just ten minutes after we parted, assuring me that it had been an unforgettable holiday and that he thought I was amazing. And now that we had finally met, he could also enjoy the pleasure of telling me something that until then I never allowed him to: he loved me.

I scolded him, despite everything, because I did not accept any compromise about this. I never wanted to hear those words until he was really convinced. I had never used them with him, for the same reason.

But Karim swore it was true, that he felt it deep in his heart. A rather new feeling, though he had had several relationships before he met me. I gave up and let those nice words accompany me for the entire trip back.

They turned and turned about in my mind, making pleasant company. And I was really in need of it.

For a change, it had started to rain since I took the highway. And for about five hundred miles it did not stop.

September 15

Once I arrived home, I immediately paid a visit to my parents. There was a visceral need to do it.

On the few times that I made a really serious mess of things, it was like I was regressing to the stage of a defenseless child and felt a pressing need for physical contact.

I had to embrace my mother and ask forgiveness for being so careless, so distracted. And then I wanted to tell her that I had been good in Germany and there was no need to worry. I would handle this new relationship as best as I could.

My mother was not there.

Or rather, she was there physically, right in front of me, but it was as if she did not live in that body anymore. Once again, she was estranged from the whole world.

Not completely, of course. She asked how the trip was and simulated a vague interest. But there was no light in the eyes and no tone in her voice.

Again lost in depression. She was going downhill at breakneck speed towards the abyss that she had faced two years earlier and from which she came back with an immense effort.

And this time as well it was all my fault.

No one else's. Only mine.

Seeing my mom in such a condition upset me, but I could never do anything for her, if she did not permit it.

My father told me that she did not want to hear about medications again. My mother never understood the critical role that they had played in her illness in the past. She did not accept the idea of using external tools, as if they represented a shame, a disgrace.

In the following days I obsessively begged my father to be near mom and not lose sight of her. I was afraid she might do something irreparable, and I could never handle it. I cursed myself a thousand times for underestimating the importance of making her part of my new story. I had excluded her from my life, and to her it represented an unacceptable insult.

She no longer felt useful to anyone.

Now that Samuele was better, and Rossella and her family had returned to their home as the big emergency was over, Mother was alone, with no opportunity to be of help. A situation that she could not accept.

In the following weeks, thanks to the medicines, things went better. My father told me that she ate regularly and slept quietly at night. I paid her a visit several times and she seemed more vital, more careful. She even went out to the grocery store and to see some friends. She was also regularly going to Mass, as she had rediscovered her faith in old age. She also involved father in her Sunday ritual: he agreed to follow her anywhere, just to see her happy.

We all breathed a sigh of relief.

And again I threw myself headlong into my long-distance relationship.

Forgetting about her, once more.

26 August 2000

Here I am, back again to express my dissatisfaction on these pages. I'm in a situation that even I can no longer understand. The relationship with Karim is getting out of hand and I do not know if one day it will still be recoverable. In recent times we just keep arguing on the phone and I am really having enough of his quirks, his paranoia.

He is more and more jealous, more possessive. Yesterday he scolded me for being alone in the shop with a male customer. Too bad it was a sixty-year-old one! A huge argument, for something so futile. Everything is becoming paradoxical and grotesque. In recent months I pretty much locked myself away in my flat, while our discussions became more insistent, more violent. Because Karim can become very harsh sometimes. When he gets mad at me, he attacks me with heavy, brutal words. I wonder whether he might be able to hurt me, if we were facing each other on these occasions. I do not even want to think about it, that's a situation I would not tolerate for anything in the world. But I cannot know, until I see him again.

In any case, when he calms down and realizes that he has exaggerated, then he humbles himself, becomes depressed, self-critical and self-destructive. He says he's not worthy of me. Sometimes he claims that without me life would not make any sense for him. Would he be capable of hurting himself?

I do not know, I do not know really.

And then he manages to bring out the worst in me, and this troubles me a lot.

Sometimes I don't even recognize myself, it's as if the one talking on the phone is a creature that was hidden inside me and that has been nourished by Karim, with his own grudge and hatred towards humanity. I do not like it at all. I'm not like that. I'm not litigious, nor polemic. I always hated to raise my voice, I've never done it with anyone before, and now I find myself shouting at the phone more and more often, exasperated.

My girlfriends are very much worried about these changes in me. They call me often, sometimes twice a day, to know how it's going. I tell them only part of my anxieties. If they knew everything, they would think it's crazy to carry on this relationship. And they would be right.

I'm allowing myself to be dragged to the bottom by a person who does not deserve me. But I have to figure out if this is the result of us living far away from each other. I need to know if living together would fix everything.

And then I'm stubborn by nature, I always have to go to the end of the road. I could never leave a trail halfway through. But if once we were together I discover that nothing has changed, then I would not have any hesitation. I would leave him immediately.

I am not afraid of solitude anymore.

I can start all over from scratch. I can find someone who does not have all these problems. I can wish for more. It is foolish to be obstinate over a lost cause. It will be tough, sure. But I have no intention of coming to terms with anybody anymore.

I did not with Jorgos. I will certainly not with Karim. Nor anyone else. Maybe one day I will come across the ideal person, or maybe not.

Well, that's all for now. See you soon and hopefully with good news!

That was the last time I wrote in my diary.

From that day on, only blank pages—as if to help erase what happened next. But no, it did not. There is no useful remedy to wipe out some events in your life. No system that works.

It would again be necessary to find the solution inside myself. It was there that I had to dig and rummage around, for the umpteenth time. Looking for new strength, new energy. Because life is a machine that needs to be fed constantly, and the fuel that is needed is not for sale anywhere. It is special. It is located in a deep well, within us.

The hardest thing is to get it out of there. But you must do it.

Sometimes it is a matter of life and death.

On September 14 my plane landed in Hamburg, Germany.

I flew there to spend a few days with Karim before we returned to Italy together. We would try to start all over again in my little apartment. He would look for a new job, and I would try to figure out if this was the man with whom I wanted to live the rest of my life.

I didn't tell anyone of my trip this time, except Rossella. I did not want my parents to worry about me or be anxious about a trip of only two or three days. I'd be home soon and they would not even notice my absence. Better for everyone.

Karim picked me up at the airport, and we spent the night in a hotel outside the city, talking about what was awaiting us in the near future. There were no unpleasant arguments, as had usually been the case, and it seemed a good step forward already. The next morning we were up late, and went out for a walk.

I was restless. For the first time in my life I was hiding a trip from my parents. I had never done it before and did not feel comfortable at all about it. I decided to call Rossella, to tell her that I was all right and perhaps I'd come back the next day. Yes, I would definitely be back the next day, because I could not last long in that guilty condition.

I dialed the number of the shop but did not find Rossella on the other end.

It was Sabrina, our shop assistant, who answered.

"Hello?" A nasal, unrecognizable voice.

"Hello, Rossella?"

Silence.

"Rossella, it's you? It's me, Cri."

"Cri..."

"Ah, Sabrina, it's you ... hi. Is Rossella in there?"

"No.... Cri ... she's not ... she just had to leave in a hurry.... Cri.... I don't know how to tell you ... something happened..." Desperate sobs.

"No. I don't want to know. I don't want to *hear* it. I'm coming back home. Come and pick me up, I'll call you from the airport."

I ran back to the hotel in a hurry, without stopping.

I had to find a flight, immediately. That was the only thing I could think of. A flight of any kind. I found one with a stopover in Paris. The only one available.

I left without a suitcase, with just the essential things. Karim would come to Italy later, bringing everything I left behind.

In Paris, the plane landed after a long delay. In terrible French, I begged the first person with a uniform that I met at the airport to help me not to miss my plane to Florence. From my eyes rather than from my words the hostess understood the drama behind my request for help. She took my hand and we ran there together, arriving just a moment before the gate closed.

Sabrina picked me up in Florence.

I arrived at my parents' house on the evening of September 15, 2000, at approximately 10:00 p.m.

There were so many people.

My two sisters.

And my father bent over a chair, his hands on his face, crying.

She gave me life.

She fed me with difficulty. She saved my life by doing this.

She spoiled me, filling me with attentions.

She put me at the center of her life, always.

She comforted me whenever there was a need.

She took care of me when I was sick.

She defended me from bad people.

She taught me how to defend myself from bad people.

She advised me in difficult times.

She stood by my side in important decisions.

She took me by the hand.

She gave me the strength that I could not find.
She held me tight, in bed, during the most terrible night ever.
She told me not to cry, that everything would be OK eventually.
She begged me to listen to her.
She implored me not to exclude her from my life.
She let me go at the end.
She loved me so much.
She loved me so much.
She loved me so much.
My mom. She was my mom.

Standby

In the following days I experienced the same feelings as after Laura's death. Every action took place as in a dream, and nothing seemed real. I behaved out of a pure spirit of inertia. I felt a huge burden in my heart.

I felt guilty, most of all. Each of us in the family was carrying a small bundle full of "ifs" and "buts." But together they constituted only a small part of the problem. I was the main cause of her defeat. I had disappointed her, pushed her away. I excluded her.

And at one point she stopped fighting. She surrendered. She decided for all of us. Courage or cowardice, value or vileness, boldness or fear, or all these things together. I would never know what had driven her to that extreme choice. I did not have the presumption to guess. And I had no right to judge.

I just knew that from then on I would never touch her, caress her, or hug her again.

She was no more, and nothing could bring her back. I would have to live with this fact forever, without being able to do anything about it.

With no right of reply.

Soon afterward I returned to live with dad. Tiziana moved to my parents' house as well, after years of living in perfect autonomy in the city. We needed each other and we had to gather together to fight the devastating pain. We were together again, a single body that would generate a greater power to try to win again. It would take some time before we got back on our feet. I was aware of that. We needed to find new energy, and that also I knew. I was back with my feet on the ground, and for the third time I had to wear the armor of inner strength that in the past had saved me from any external attack.

In this new state of affairs there could be no room for Karim.

A few weeks after his arrival in Italy, I told him that it would not be possible to carry on the relationship. I had other priorities—much more important ones.

He protested, got angry, calmed down, finally humbled himself again. He bombarded me with text messages and calls for another month. And eventually he surrendered. He left my apartment in December, and I had no desire whatsoever to know his destination.

A closed chapter, double-locked.

In December, on the last day of that disastrous year, my father discovered that he had bladder cancer.

Throughout his life, until then, he had suffered only the occasional cold. Now it was as if he had given up and did not want to live anymore, he and his body with him. Seven years later, the disease would have the better of that energetic, vital man. But in that first phase, fortunately, surgery and a few days of hospitalization led to a very quick recovery. And, according to Rossella's theory of the half-full glass, the disease served to shake Dad out of the apathy that had trapped him in the house since Mom had gone.

My father had finally begun to live because he realized that it could still be an interesting thing to do. After a few months he urged Tiziana and me to return to our homes. He would manage by himself.

And so, in March of 2001, I moved back to my apartment.

After emptying the suitcases I sat down on the bed with an absent look. I sighed, tired, then I closed my eyes for a second and when I opened them again my attention settled on an object. One that had caused a fair share of turmoil in my recent life experience, but, if used reasonably, one that might still reveal some pleasant surprises.

If only I had a little luck, if only the wheel would come to rest on my number—

This time I would be careful. I would notice any negative signal and run for cover promptly. I would read between the lines, carefully, and understand, because now I realized the destructive power that it could hide. Despite everything I would try again, with extreme caution. I would turn it on and give myself another chance.

I was sure it would all be all right.

This time it would be my friend, because for me it was, after all, a friend.

It had kept me company for many evenings, made me laugh and thrilled me. It had been a traveling companion.

And it was still there, still in its place.
On hold. On standby.

Maya

This time I would not start out in a chat room.

I did not want to go over paths already beaten in the past and which reminded me only of bad feelings. On television, almost by accident, I noticed the ad for a new online dating site. Its icon was a puppy dog surrounded by a heart. I registered on it just for fun, to see how such a thing worked. In the initial questionnaire I filled some fields that would tell the world my personal tastes in books, music, movies and sports, and above all my hatred for any physical activity that involved lifting more than one finger at a time. I was lazy, and I absolutely had to communicate that as the very first bit of information.

As a final step, it was necessary to write an introductory message, a kind of personal presentation, that all users could read on my profile page. I read a few and noticed that many users described themselves with far too many adjectives and attributes only vaguely related to reality. After all, who could ever find out otherwise or refute those claims?

I, on the other hand, was not going to reveal too much of myself.

I would remain vague, just to spice the whole situation up a bit.

I chose a new nickname. Enough with the past. No more names derived from stupid ideas of retaliation.

I had recently met a very sweet Hungarian girl, thanks to my Budapest-based friend Iko, one of the people who had been closest to me since we first met, fifteen years earlier, during a twinship of our respective high schools.

From the beginning of our friendship, Iko had always understood everything about my feelings, my insecurities, and me. She had a special relationship with me and in time a very strong bond formed between us. Although she lived in Budapest, we met on a regular basis, every year, and were constantly in touch through close correspondence.

A beautiful, priceless relationship. A friendship that went beyond long distance and any kind of physical boundaries.

In those early days of March, I was returning from one such trip to Hungary and felt loads of energy in me, just like every time we met.

Iko had introduced me to a new female friend. Maya. A beautiful name, and a perfect one for me to steal and make it "virtually" mine.

On Tuesday, March 6, 2001, Maya (@ 989 496) published the following announcement: "Well.... What to say so as not to seem banal? Maybe just avoid saying anything.... And if anyone will ever be intrigued by this tiny little message.... Well.... I am here! It seems so strange to use a medium this ... strange.... But life is full of surprises.... And who knows..."

A lot of ellipses and suspension points. A whole lot. But I liked it. The tiny little message, as I had called it, sounded at least a bit interesting and unusual. With those words I hoped to draw the attention of interesting and unusual people. Would I be successful in my aims?

Well ... who knows ...

I went to bed and immediately forgot all about it. Too many thoughts in my head, still confused and unresolved.

The next day I did not turn on the computer. Not even in the next two days. I completely ignored the idea of having received any response to my tiny little message.

On the evening of March 9, I finally checked my e-mail. Much to my surprise, there were sixty-four unread messages, all from the online dating site. I could not believe my eyes. I started laughing like crazy, in the silence of my room. I was enjoying this new game a whole lot.

It took me all night to read them. I finished at five in the morning, but I had spent several extraordinary hours. Some messages were short, insignificant. Others resembled those texts of introduction to the site, all the same, full of redundant adjectives and not very credible. But some messages were really intriguing. One in particular struck me very much for the grammatical correctness, the use of terms, the punctuation.

Fussy as I had always been, a sympathizer and supporter of the use of ellipses as well as the right term in the right place, I just loved those details. Furthermore, it was a letter that spoke, and told interesting stories.

I was fascinated. More. I was captured. Kidnapped.

That message had travelled from the Northern city of Parma right here to me, in my room in a village in the Tuscan countryside. And it made the difference, in the end it really made the difference. That night, events began to occur in an incredibly fast way, heading without delay towards that happy ending that I had wanted so much throughout my life.

On the night of March 10, I replied to that first message. Other e-mails followed, more and more intimate, emphatic, engaging.

Then, on 15 March 2001, we spoke on the phone for the first time. We talked for a whole night.

On March 24, Roberto came over to see me. On May 1 I introduced him to my family. That September I went to Parma to meet his parents. In December we spent Christmas with his family and New Year's Day with his friends. Immediately after the holidays Rob left his city and moved to my house. On June 23, 2002, we got married.

It was not the best day of my life. It would be unfair to say that.

It was a special moment, of course. But every day with him has been unique, exclusive and unrepeatable. From first to last. To choose the happiest would be too complicated. A venture as useless as impossible.

Rob means everything to me. And I to him.

We never spend a day without remembering to ourselves how lucky we were to meet each other. He has filled my life with joy, passion, peace, respect, sharing. He has made me laugh, moved me, and thrilled me. He has enriched my culture, teaching me millions of things I did not know. He has understood me beyond any imagination.

He has completed me.

And most of all he has loved me for what I am.

I could go on for hours, telling how much Rob has made my life incredibly happy, my dear Nancy, but I guess you get the idea. We are the two halves of the Platonic myth who met after looking for each other their whole lives.

I have only one regret. If I had known my husband a year, or only a few months earlier, my family would all still here with us. I am sure.

My mom would have realized that he represents everything I ever searched for, and she would have been happy. She would have spent with us so many more years, having her happiness back at last. And my father with her.

Or maybe not. Maybe their sacrifice was necessary for me to take a new path. To turn the page, one last time.

I don't know. I really don't know.

23 June 2002. One of the happiest days of my life.

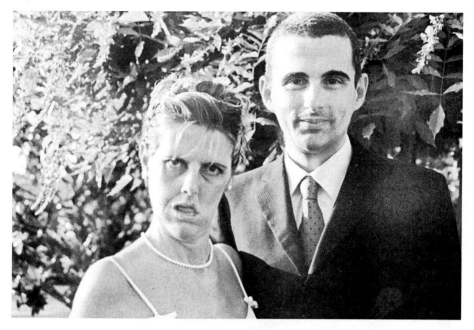

23 June 2002. On the day of my wedding with my love, Roberto.

One thing is certain: my life has been a race, a path full of obstacles. But the ultimate prize I received is an enormous love whose power has healed all the wounds, dried all the tears, and erased all the pain.

I could never ask for more than I have been given.

Rob is a precious gift.

The most important of all.

Rob is my life.

To Be and Not to Be (Able to...)

There are things that I am not able to do because of the syndrome. Attitudes, expressions, social relationships that I have been denied. For each of them, I have always searched for a ploy, a way to get around the problem, sometimes succeeding, sometimes not.

But it has always been important to *try*.

(1) I cannot chew.

Many people with Moebius Syndrome, almost all of them, have this capacity, whereas I lack the nerve designed for this task. A *rarity* within the *rarity*. The solution to this problem was obvious and immediate. As soon as I was able to use my hands knowledgeably, I immediately began to employ them to facilitate the act of chewing by putting one under the chin and pushing it upwards so as to support the movement of the jaw. And if one was not enough, I used both.

Nothing fancy. Just a little embarrassing for an outside observer who, not knowing my congenital difficulties, might think themselves in front of a rather strange chick who does not even have good table manners. In time—very soon, actually—I learned to lose interest in the cartoon thought bubbles I could feel hovering over the heads of those who watched me eat. It was a simple matter of survival: either eat in front of strangers without being ashamed of the strange method I had to employ or starve.

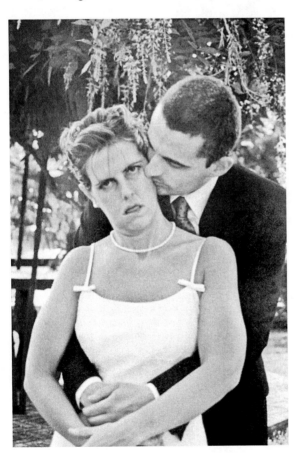

23 June 2002. Roberto and I posing for the wedding photographs.

Still, at the beginning, even though I was just a little girl with no social conscience, I did have some trouble with that. In kindergarten, for one, I had a terrible time: as soon as I sat together with the other children for lunch, I felt nauseous and could not eat anything. The worried teachers reported my by now daily lack of appetite to my mother, who in turn worried a lot, but wisely decided to feed me in a more substantial way at home, saving me unnecessary and harmful guilt.

After a few months, the problem disappeared completely. With hindsight, it is very likely that I had suffered a shock at the first meal with my peers. Maybe some kid had made an inappropriate comment seeing me eat in a very peculiar way and this had inhibited my desire for food. Or maybe some other unconscious mechanism had clicked. The fact is that after passing that first difficult confrontation with the normal community, I have not felt ashamed to eat in front of anyone.

And if said outside observer just cannot stand the sight of me chewing, that's his own problem: he may as well turn the other way. Enjoying a good meal is something too important to be disturbed by people's ignorance.

(2) I cannot take a bite of a sandwich.

A small footnote to point number one, but a bit more complicated to solve, especially if the sandwich belongs to someone else. A hundred, a thousand times at school, during mid-morning breaks, some gentle soul generously offered me to taste their oh-so-inviting sandwich, which almost always aroused in me an irresistible desire to bite into it without missing a second. But, just as many times I had to politely refuse. I could not afford to take a bite from my own sandwich, let alone someone else's.

For breakfast I rarely brought a sandwich as most of my companions did, since I was well aware that biting my way into it would be impossible. Yet I would have liked to, and how! At most, I could tear off small pieces with my hands, but it was a torture to both the poor, hapless sandwich and me, so I almost always avoided doing it. Especially since managing that small and hostile piece of bread and being confronted by so many curious glances required a superhuman effort. My hands were already engaged in holding the object of my desire, and I could not use them to help me in chewing.

In short, it was an enterprise worthy of a fearless hero. And I did not feel like that at all.

So, in this case, the solution to the problem has always been to get around it a priori. Soft snacks, yogurt, fruits, Mom's pies could be substitutes just as delicious.

Nevertheless, I still have an exaggerated love for sandwiches. Almost mystical, I would say.

(3) I cannot suck from a straw.

Weird problem, seemingly innocuous, but one that still manages to irritate me. I cannot close my lips around the damn straw.

Unless ... I position the drink on the table, gather the fingers of both hands around the lips so as to close them forcibly around the straw and at that point suck up the contents of the glass-can-bottle-whatever. Ugly to look at, again, from the outside, but as I said before, who cares.

Learning to ignore other people's reactions in this case required a bit of extra work, but in the end my pride got the better of me, and when it is necessary I have no problem in using the evil suction tool. Especially in the case of gaily colored contraptions with strange shapes, fitted with endless roundabouts and vortices. Irresistible!

And let others have a good look, while I enjoy my delicious cocktail without any inhibition. Moreover (see point number one), you are always free to turn your head the other way, in any democratic country in the world, if you don't like the show. Or am I wrong?

(4) I cannot go scuba diving.

The mouthpiece: that insidious, undefeated enemy. I could write a book about it.

Never, never, never have I managed to get the better of that dreadful device, a thousand times worse than the terrible but eventually tamable straw. With the mouthpiece there is no outside help that works. I could use one, two, a hundred hands, but I would never be able to close my lips completely around it. And in this case, even if only a trickle of water passes inside the breathing tube—well, you can imagine the rest.

Every summer I tried tirelessly to use the mouthpiece in safe waters, knowing that it would cause me at least five minutes of a choking cough, aggravated by the horrible taste of the ingested salty water. But as always I did not want to give up. Then, one summer, having risked drowning, I decided that maybe it was best to give up and concede to the mouthpiece the honor of undisputed victory. A devastating defeat for my ego, one of the rare occasions when I found no solutions whatsoever. Difficult to accept, but sometimes you have to admit the impossibility of being able to succeed in everything.

No diving, then. But there is nothing that can stop me from snorkeling: only mask, fins and the ability to hold my breath for as long as possible. And I have become very good over the years. Watching the small fish that live near the surface, so numerous as to satisfy my innate curiosity, is more than enough for me, thank goodness.

(5) I cannot whistle.

Too bad. Sometimes I would just love to draw the attention of some nice-looking guy passing by. Or maybe not. You know, Nancy, I don't think my husband would be particularly happy with that. And then, let's face it, I always found whistling a rather vulgar act, and I do not think it is simply a case of the fox and the grapes syndrome.

Whistling is not suitable for gentle, polite young ladies. I was one once. A young lady, I mean. Gentle and polite.

That's why, now that I'm not like that anymore, I sometimes fancy experimenting with new whistling methods. As you must have realized by now, I cannot stand the idea of not being able to do something, even if that something is a somewhat questionable sound.

With whistling I had to do it my way as well.

The method I learned first allows me to issue a nice powerful whistle: I squeeze my lower lip between the thumb and forefinger and suck up the air so as to obtain the desired effect. Powerful but inelegant, if there is such a thing as an "elegant whistle."

Then there is another system I learned recently on a day that I did not have any specific mental and physical commitments and time to devote to such highly useful experiments. With the help of the thumb and forefinger, but this time using both hands, I join the lips, protracting them in the usual way that allows one to blow a whistle, and exhale. The first attempts were a disaster, I admit. I expelled large amounts of air, but no sound whatsoever. But since I am the stubborn type, I finally managed to modulate a note, only one, which over time evolved into a melodic sound. A few tones high and low, nothing special, but a great result from my particular point of view, after years of one-note whistles.

The last method, equal to the second in execution, consists of inhaling air instead of exhaling it. You will not believe it, but this way I am able to emit modulated sounds. And with great satisfaction. Sure—thin, delicate, fragile—but still melodic.

After all this elaborate explanation I would not want to make you think, dear Nancy, that I delight myself in the fine art of whistling. Sometimes, however, it might be useful and, as my father would have said, it's good to have something to fall back on, just in case.

(6) I cannot blow.

Which is often translated as: I cannot blow out the candles of a birthday cake.

Well, I found a little trick again, in this case bringing the tongue to the upper lip (the lower one being unusable), but the result is a very feeble breeze, capable of extinguishing just the few closest candles at most. OK for the first birthdays. The problem gradually amplified as the number of candles on the cake grew. At about fifteen years old I began to worry seriously about never being able to fulfill any of my wishes: I was now hopelessly unable to extinguish them in one fell swoop. A serious problem, very serious.

Then, progress and marketing came to my aid.

Until puberty I had to make do with only the classic birthday cake candles, pink and serpentine-shaped. Then some genius, never amply rewarded for so much initiative, invented a candle in the shape of a number, saving at one stroke my fragile teenage mental balance and possibly a bad impression in front of dozens of guests.

Finally, in the future I would have only two candles to blow out, which changed from year to year, but always only two. My wishes were safe.

Praise to you, O unknown inventor.

(7) I cannot inflate balloons.

In Bulgaria, in the year 1992, I felt lost because of this shortcoming. I was traveling with my then-boyfriend in my tireless Lancia Ypsilon 10. We left Greece and drove for about 15 uninterrupted hours to Italy following a well-planned program: a few stops, no time to rest, alternating driving, a little doze for each of us while on the "navigator" shift.

As a result, I was driving, in the middle of an Eastern bloc country, with a pair of red eyes that would make a zombie proud. Then, of course, came a checkpoint. The policeman approaches, does not speak or understand any language but his own, directs me impatiently to get out of the car and hands me a device. I recognize it with horror. A breath alcohol tester with an inflatable balloon.

I spend the next ten minutes trying to explain to the police officer, in all the languages I know, that it's not that I don't want to—fact is, I just can't blow up the damn balloon.

Non posso. Je ne peux pas. No puedo. Ich kann nicht. Den mporò. I cannot!

Simultaneously I gesticulate wildly, pointing at my lips, my face, and my handicap. He doesn't look moved, not the least bit. He looks askance and keeps pointing at the device. In desperation I begin to walk a straight imaginary line, arms open wide, one foot behind the other, in the classic way that serves to demonstrate lucidity and sobriety.

No use. He remains impassive. Indeed, he gets nervous. I, on the other hand, am starting to panic. Then, the stroke of genius, the divine illumination. I remember having several cans of Coke behind the seat. Cigarettes they are not, that's true, but it is a product of great Western civilization. And it works. The Coca-Cola Company saved us.

Nevertheless, after so many years, I still cannot blow up balloons of any kind. And so I have no solution for this very problem. I just have to hope I come across an Italian policeman next time.

Oh, by the way, I'm a teetotaler.

(8) I cannot smoke.

I never really suffered for this, to tell you the truth. The fact that I could not join my lips and breathe in a substance that most probably would bring me nothing but health issues never troubled me that much. Indeed, it led me to think over and over again that I was quite lucky, since I could not fall into temptation.

Sure, in the critical high school years, in the endless moments of discomfort when I did not know how to show disdain, it would have been helpful to have a cigarette between my fingers. It would have symbolized my indifference to the community of people who at parties, in nightclubs, or in any other social gathering did not deign to look at me. A cigarette would have given me strength, deluded me that I placed a barrier between the outside world and myself. But no, I could not. And I did not want to.

If twenty years ago mobile phones had existed, they would have saved me every single moment of embarrassment: those of you who have never pretended to fiddle on the keyboard so as not to seem in distress, raise your hand.

I do it often. If I don't want to be disturbed, for example. Or if I am momentarily alone at a restaurant table. Or if I'm waiting for someone who is late. Moments of solitude that nothing and no one could fill better than a smartphone or a cigarette. Today, I can at least take advantage of the former (which, not coincidentally, is *smart*). In the eighties I couldn't.

My moments of solitude in crowded places were spent in counting the seconds, hoping they would end as soon as possible, but without any outside help. Sometimes I formulated a wish: a divine intervention that turned me invisible or magic that made all the others disappear in one fell swoop.

Certainly, however, I never relied on cigarettes to dispel embarrassment. I have always been very proud of that and I will continue to be so.

(9) I cannot blow raspberries.

Frustrating, in some cases. But acceptable. I never looked for alternative solutions.

In return I can make enviable bigmouths.

(10) I cannot do a passable Angelina Jolie impersonation.

I made up my mind to do it, even if I had to work it out a bit. It was not easy to give up.

A New Family

Alice was staring at me, her eyes still bright with tears.

Her parents had approached me a few minutes earlier and confessed that I had touched her in a profound way. She ran away in the car after hearing my story, unable to resist the emotions that overran like a flooding river.

Alice was 18 years old, still too young to fight against such powerful, sudden, unexpected feelings. She had listened to my presentation at the National Congress of the Italian Moebius Syndrome Association, where I told my story: a few pages where I summarized forty years of life and my own experience with the syndrome.

I was asked to share my experiences with all the other families who had to deal every day with the same difficulties I had gone through, and I gladly agreed. Maybe I could kindle hope in them. Maybe my own happy ending, my having found a way beyond the darkness of adolescence, could rejuvenate some sensitive, still fragile soul.

Like Alice.

Alice joined us out of the conference room, after she calmed down. She was still struggling to fight back the tears. But it was better. As I told the story of my life, she felt as if my words somehow belonged to her as well. And I was developing feelings very similar to hers.

To be there, in front of her, was like watching myself reflected in a mirror. Another Cristina, once again a little girl, frail and defenseless.

Yes, I had been there too.

I perfectly understood the avalanche of feelings that were devouring her. Alice was going through the most difficult period: the flurry of adolescence, that dramatic moment when you think that no one cares about you and your life will be just a set of unhappy days, one after the other.

Meeting Alice broke my heart.

I tried to console her. I told her that what she was going through was just a phase. The most painful one. Then life would give her unimaginable possibilities.

I told her how easy it had been for me to communicate through a medium that allowed me to display my soul first, whereas my physical aspect came afterwards. She could use a computer too, but with care and common sense, because it might also become too dangerous a weapon. I assured Alice that there would be a Rob somewhere, soon, very soon, for her too. She just needed a little patience and all would be well.

But then I stopped.

I thought that, after all, every story is unique and unrepeatable. I could not convey the strength I had gained over the years to that delicate little girl. I had built it day by day, obstacle after obstacle, along my way. Alice would have her own path, a path more or less difficult, which she would have to face with her own strength, and no one else's.

She would decide whether to move forward or stop.

I could give her only a glimmer of hope, nothing else.

But it was enough.

Alice eventually took my hands in hers and whispered something, looking into my eyes.

Thank you.

The first time I typed on a search engine the words "Moebius Syndrome" was in 2000, shortly after buying my first PC and entering the magical world of the World Wide Web. I did not expect to find much information about it.

And yet almost immediately I came across the site created by Renzo De Grandi, the father of a little girl suffering from the syndrome and who at that time was putting together A.I.S.Mo. (Associazione Italiana Sindrome di Moebius, or Italian Moebius Syndrome Association), a nonprofit association, to try to bring public attention to this very rare disease: the incidence of the Moebius Syndrome is about 1 in 1 million.

Through that Web site, I learnt much more about the disease, and the more I read, the more I realized how lucky I was compared to many others. In addition to the most significant element—the lack of facial expression—the syndrome might also cause many other issues: difficulty in eating and swallowing, with even the risk of choking; hypersensitivity of the eyes (which, since the eyelids are not able to close completely, are often bloodshot); absence of lateral movements of the eyes; strabismus; limited movement of the tongue; hearing loss. There could even be additional features such as weak muscle tone, as well as abnormalities in the hands and feet, such as clubfeet or missing fingers or toes.

Renzo took his little daughter up to Canada to meet the only professor in the world who was studying this issue. I already knew that name. I had heard it one day, by sheer chance, watching the news a few years earlier. Dr. Ronald Zuker.

On that TV report there was talk of an American girl, Chelsey Thomas, who suffered from a rare disease that, since birth, had prevented her from smiling. That child had been successfully operated on by a team of Canadian doctors and had finally found her smile. There had been no particular mention of any syndrome. It was typical broadcasting news stuff, generic and conceived so as to be understandable to a wide audience. But I quickly realized that it was about my problem: that news report spoke of me, of my *rarity*.

In 1997, the Internet was still unknown to me. I was not even aware that such a system of global communication existed. But that didn't stop me. After the broadcast ended, I immediately looked for a phone number and called the TV channel. The switchboard passed my call to the news editorial staff, and there I finally got to speak with the author of the report that had so interested me.

The journalist was very kind. She understood that it was the first time, after twenty-seven years of living with the syndrome, that I had come across a story like that. Until that time, in spite of everything, I was still convinced that I was almost unique in the world. The journalist gave me the name of the Canadian professor and the addresses that she had obtained during the making of the report. I wrote everything in a diary, but in the end I put aside the notion of flying to Canada to solve my problems. The idea of such a difficult journey scared me, for so many different reasons, almost as if it were an unattainable mirage.

But Renzo, a few years later, had that courage.

He took his little girl, Giulia, to Dr. Zuker, getting there by different routes, most likely. Certainly the Internet was the new medium that marked a turning point in his research. Without imagining it, Renzo had embarked on that journey of hope on my behalf, as well as for all those families who still didn't know that a solution finally existed.

After reading Giulia's story on the Web site I had found and in some newspaper articles that had reported on it, I wrote an e-mail to the Italian Moebius Syndrome Association, telling of my own experience in a few simple lines. There was no need for many words to express the feelings that overwhelmed me after discovering its existence. Like so many others, I had been searching for some support, a reference point, for a whole lifetime. And now I had found it.

Renzo answered enthusiastically. He was grateful that I had come forward. He explained that many cases and many families were still wandering in a limbo of ignorance, not knowing that there was finally an association to rely on. Every time a new member of that small, unusual community manifested itself, coming out of anonymity, it was a joy.

From that day on I would no longer feel alone. I was part of a larger family, made up of people like me. I had finally shrugged that tremendous word off my shoulders.

It had accompanied me for many years, but now it did not scare me anymore.

A horrible term, but harmless by now.

Rarity.

Over the years, inquiring through the association, I discovered that in Italy there were dozens of families affected by Moebius Syndrome, each with a story to tell, like mine.

A few years after its birth, the association organized a meeting, a first national congress, to try to take stock of the situation. Up to that point Renzo had never stopped. He had gathered a team of doctors and surgeons and made sure they would go to Canada and learn from Dr. Zuker how to perform the "smile surgery," so as to introduce it to Italy as well.

I wanted to go to that meeting, but on the other hand I was extremely hesitant. I talked to Rob about it, and he persuaded me to attend.

But I was anxious.

I was worried about meeting people who had the same problem, as if that confrontation might deprive me of my uniqueness, a feeling hard to explain, and one which bothered me a lot.

In the end we attended the congress and enjoyed an experience of disarming intensity. There were tears and laughter and a variety of indescribable emotions.

A boy suffering from the syndrome told his story, and several times, as he read, I immersed myself completely in his words, as if they were my own. Two lives so far apart and yet so similar. He generated an enormous sense of empathy in my heart, like a brother I met only that day for the first time.

A disarming, inexplicable feeling.

Unbelievable.

During the convention I was also able to meet Dr. Ronald Zuker, an event which a few years earlier had seemed an impossibility. The Canadian professor studied my case and told me that he could not operate on me successfully.

I constituted a *rarity* within the *rarity*: I was lacking a vital facial nerve that was needed in order to connect the muscle graft from the thigh and activate the much-desired smile. Therefore, it was impossible, in my case, to achieve any significant result.

The news did not sadden me. In fact, I was almost relieved. I thought I would not be able to make up my mind if I had been given another chance. I was now 36 years old, had a husband who adored me and so much self-confidence accumulated over the years. Enough to make me aware of being a *normal* person, like anyone else, even if a bit special.

My path of awareness and acceptance was complete. Better this way. I would be myself for the rest of my life.

Five years have passed since that day.

I attended a second congress held by the association, where I met Alice. I underwent two medical examinations at the hospital in Parma, the only center in Italy where the "smile surgery" is performed. A most amazing coincidence indeed, given that Parma is also the city where my husband was born and lived until our paths crossed.

There, the surgeon who examined me, Dr. Bernardo Bianchi, told me that there was a new chance. On both occasions, a year after each other, he confirmed that he would be able to operate on me. To make up for the lack of the nerve (the fourth facial nerve, the one used for chewing) that is employed to connect the grafted muscle, he would use a nerve from my shoulder, pulling it back and attaching it to the gracilis muscle taken from the thigh. A bit more complicated than usual, nevertheless it was possible.

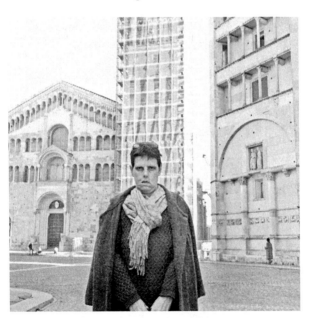

Taking a walk in the cathedral square in Parma, on the day before undergoing smile surgery. I have never been so scared in my life.

The news disturbed me a bit. Actually, a lot. By now, I had accepted the fact that I would never be able to smile. Let bygones be bygones. And now that it seemed possible, did I really want it?

I was terrified that a surgical intervention might change the situation and affect mechanisms that were now my own from an entire life. So delicate and fragile—and at the same time well tested and effective.

Speaking, for example. Could I still use the same method when pronouncing labials? Or would I have to start from scratch and practice in using both lips instead of the tongue? How long would it take to learn a whole new system? And would I be able, at forty years of age, to put everything back into the game?

I thought about it.

One year.

Then a few more months.

And a few more days. And finally I decided: I had to do it.

Because you can never be content with what you have.

Because you should always aspire to something better.

Because if life pushes you back into the game, you cannot pretend nothing has happened.

Because my parents had spent years looking for this kind of response.

Because now that it's within my reach it would be a shame to ignore it.

Because it would be cowardly and unjust not to try.

Because you have to keep fighting. Always.

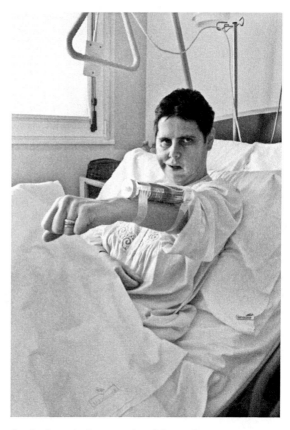

At the hospital, a couple of days after surgery, I proudly show the syringe-attached anesthetic dispenser (which actually reminded me of those lethal weapons in sci-fi flicks).

In 1985 I underwent plastic surgery to please my parents. In 1993 I underwent another to please my then-boyfriend and his family. This time I decided to do it for myself. Because I deserved it and that is that.

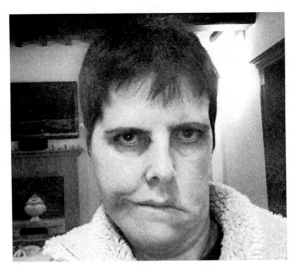

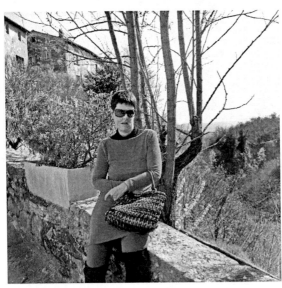

Top: **December 2013. One month after undergoing the smile surgery in Parma. The transplanted muscle still has to fully relax.** *Bottom:* **Spring 2014. In the countryside near Cortona.**

I have been told not to harbor high hopes. I have been told that there are no guarantees of success. And I'm scared, so scared. But if I gave up this last game with the syndrome, I would not have any respect for myself anymore. And no, I could not just stand it. One last game.

Or, as they say in Greece, *To teleftèo pechnìdi.*

And so here I am, Nancy, in this hospital bed, ready to give a new twist to my life. I'm still sleepy because of the anesthesia and I don't feel like waking up completely.

You ask me to open my eyes, but I would like to wait a little longer. It feels so good in this kind of limbo, in this comfortable nest. In this cocoon.

There is peace and quiet here. I would love to stay longer in this postoperative numbness. You know that I'm lazy, I told you, didn't I?

But I cannot allow myself too much time. I

am here to win yet another battle against the syndrome. Probably the mother of all battles.

Our personal dispute began over 40 years ago, and it seems that She, the syndrome, does not want to give up—ever.

She wants to have the last word on everything and direct my life as it pleases Her best. And as much as I try, She always comes back, each time stronger than before. She seems to make fun of me.

I should hate Her, despise Her, loathe Her with all my strength.

And yet I don't. Absolutely not.

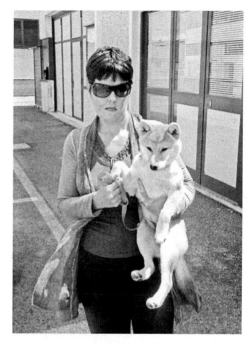

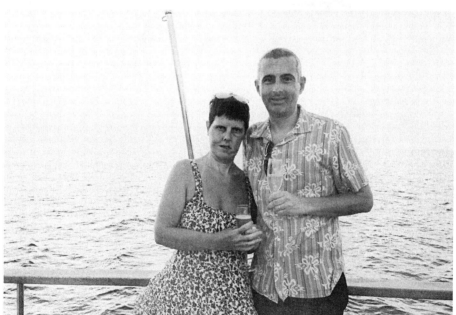

Top: Summer 2014. With my Shiba dog Maya. *Bottom:* December 2014. A smile from the Maldives islands!

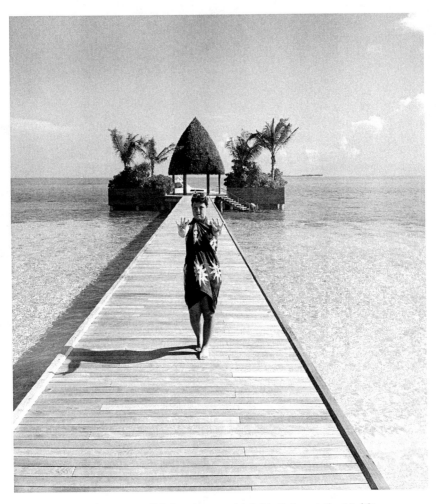

5 December 2014. Celebrating my 44th birthday at the Maldives.

In time I came to realize that the syndrome has saved me, by giving me a full life, which I would never have had a chance to live otherwise. A life all uphill, yet intense, full of deep emotions, and lived with every fiber of my being.

The syndrome has made me become the person I am. She pushed me to have confidence in myself. She gave me strength, determination, stubbornness. She deleted my insecurities and turned them into certainties. She made sure that I blossomed and was born to a new life.

And now that I'm here, there is no time to be lazy. There are still so many things to do, and a whole life to live. And millions of smiles to give.

You are right, Nancy. I will listen to you. I have to open my eyes. It is time to get out of this warm and welcoming cocoon. Now it is time to fly.

Like a small butterfly.

San Mikrí Petalùda.

Index

Numbers in *bold italics* indicate pages with photographs.